M000305402

Inner Radiance, Outer Beauty

by Ambika Wauters

THE CROSSING PRESS
FREEDOM, CALIFORNIA

Copyright © 2001 by Ambika Wauters
Cover design by Victoria May
Cover photograph © Daniel E. Arsenault/Imagebank
Interior design by Courtnay Perry
Printed in the U.S.A.

For information on bulk purchases or group discounts for this and other Crossing Press titles, please contact our Special Sales Manager at 800/777-1048.

Visit our Web site: **www.crossingpress.com**

Library of Congress Cataloging-in-Publication Data

Wauters, Ambika.
    Inner radiance, outer beauty / by Ambika Wauters.
        p. cm.
    Includes bibliographical references.
    ISBN 1-58091-080-7 (pbk.)
    1. Beauty, Personal. 2. Meditations. 3. Health. I. Title.

RA778 .W226 2001
646.7--dc21

00-064434

Acknowledgments

I would like to acknowledge the following people for their help and assistance in completing this book. To Eva Chrysanthou and her family, who run the Sulphur Springs Hotel in the village of Miliou, near Phapos, Cyprus, where I stayed while writing this book. Sincere thanks to the management of the Coral Beach Hotel in Coral Bay, Cyprus, for allowing me access to their Health and Beauty Spa. Thanks to Eva Maratheftiou, Ziba Dionysiou, Stella Pelivanidou, Maria Kyriakou, Athy Makriou, and Christine Athanasiou for their professional expertise in beauty care management. Thanks to the staff of the Enchantment Resort in Sedona, Arizona, who helped me with research. Thanks to Elaine Gill of The Crossing Press for her support of this book. And to the healers, therapists, and beauticians who helped me understand and cultivate my own unique sense of beauty.

This book is dedicated to the truly beautiful people I have known in my life. Their beauty reflected a warm and loving heart, goodness of character, and a confirmed sense of their worth. They shine in my memory because their beauty embraced me and made me feel loved and cherished and, indeed, beautiful. As always, my grandmother, Essie Ferer, taught me the healing power of unconditional love. She remained beautiful to all who loved her well into her late 80s. She was stunning, elegant, and beautiful to the core of her being. She helped me realize one of my tasks in life is to make the world a more beautiful place for us all.

Table of Contents

Age cannot wither her, nor custom stale her infinite variety; other women cloy the appetites they feed, but she makes hungry where most she satisfies…

—Shakespeare, *Antony and Cleopatra*

Introduction

My life is rich in experience and adventures, yet I age just like everyone else, and like everyone else, I wonder what I can do to maintain and enhance my looks. In exploring my attitudes about my looks I realize I have had a fixed vision of myself for most of my life. I have liked my eyes, disliked my thighs and legs, wondered what on earth I could do about my wild, curly hair, and fretted about skin blemishes, facial hair, and flabby upper arms. I don't think that I am different from millions of other women my age. It's a universal phenomenon we all experience.

I have never had conventional looks, shape, or thoughts by anyone's standard. Nor could I measure up to a fashion magazine's definition of beauty, no matter how hard I tried. Hoping for help, I bought countless bottles and jars of cosmetics and creams and have been disappointed time and again by the results. So I decided to do some research into the subject of beauty. Through the work, I came to understand that the way I looked was the result of my beliefs and attitudes. On the basis of that research, I realized that I needed to create a new model or template that would support my growing sense of self-worth as I aged and matured.

Over the years in my workshops, I noticed that when women began to believe in themselves and experienced their potential for beauty, they blossomed. They created a template of intent that changed the way they looked and felt about themselves. It's truly amazing to see how different women look when they start the process of loving and honoring themselves.

If we believe that we are ugly and no one loves us, no matter what we do to ourselves (including putting the knife to our faces or having our thighs pumped free of fat), nothing will change our underlying and self-fulfilling lack of faith in ourselves. The world always mirrors back our inner truth about our selves.

If we want to be beautiful, it is necessary to create the inner template for that to happen. If we do not do the necessary inner work, and if we sit around waiting for Prince Charming (and we all have the fantasy that he is out there, he's the *one*, right?) to drive up and fall over when he sees how lovely and wonderful we are, we are deluding ourselves. We are placing the responsibility for empowerment outside of ourselves. And no matter how drop-dead gorgeous he is, eventually we will want to reclaim our own power and energy.

It is up to us to create ourselves in the image we want to be, including how we look and how we feel. If we have an idea that beauty is cold, tight, and exclusive, as it appears in the fashion journals, we are truly going to suffer. People may admire us, but who in the world would want to hug us? Besides, who can love a carbon copy?

I have taken this quest from loving myself on the inside to its natural conclusion of loving myself on the outside, and looking at the products, hair styles, and makeup that can enhance my appearance. Love the inside and reflect it on the outside is my code. I began this process by visualizing the possibilities and working on what needed enhancing: my body, my diet, and my spiritual connection with the Source, as well as skin care, makeup, and hair style. In my experience, all of these create the effect of health and beauty. Beauty is not meant to be an aspect of the ego. It is, in truth, the fulfillment of our physical, emotional, and spiritual potential.

Please note I am not talking about narcissism when I suggest that we tap into our potential for beauty and grace. I am speaking about a non-ego awareness of our bodies and our appearance that can express our inner light. Why keep all that spiritual beauty under wraps? Who will get to share in it? When real beauty emerges, it astounds us and whoever meets us. It is a real gift, meant to be shared.

Beauty is not the exclusive property of the young and slim. It is the birthright of every person. You may have to do the work to bring that beauty out to the surface, but what gift of God doesn't require some work to reach its potential?

This book was written in Cyprus, the birthplace of Aphrodite, the goddess of love and beauty. Cypriot mythology holds that every woman has the potential to become Aphrodite. This book is designed to help you manifest the goddess of beauty within you and to help you release those old punishing regimes many women follow. It can encourage you to find your own path to inner acceptance and beauty.

I wish you well on your path. May you always know your beauty and your worth.

Part I

Inner Beauty:
Seeking the Self

Chapter 1

℘Opening to the Higher Self

Beauty is luminescence and radiance. It can be measured in the timbre of your voice, and the way you move your body and hold your spine. It is seen in the warmth of your smile and the joy and openness of your embrace. When you meet someone beautiful, there is no one thing you can identify as beautiful to the exclusion of something else. Yet, you can't make someone beautiful with all the surgery, treatments, or cosmetics. In the realm of the Self, that part of our being that is one with Infinite Intelligence and Universal Love is an aspect of our soul's worth. Some call this God, others call it the Christ Light—still others relate it to the One we are all connected to. It has many names. At this core level beauty is who we are. It is our Self.

This inner Self is where you will find the light, love, freedom, and the goodness you desire. These qualities are immutable and come with the territory of your humanity. They are part of each individual soul and there is nothing you have to do to achieve them. These qualities are within you.

We can connect with the Self through meditation and prayer

and begin the process of releasing neurotic, petty concerns about how we look. At that point we begin to know that beauty is an intrinsic part of who we are, and this helps us redefine ourselves in a new light.

Opening to this place within creates the foundation from which our beauty and grace can be accessed. Translating that aspect of ourselves into a kinetic, living reality then becomes a choice, as well as a statement of inner awareness. Out of this connection with the Higher Self we can formulate a new archetype or model of beauty which is not defined by external reality, but is anchored in our inner awareness. This is inner work we must each do for ourselves. Making this connection implies we are willing to be the best that we can be. The more we affirm our worth, the stronger and more empowered this archetype becomes and the more our inner beauty radiates into the world.

The peace we experience from this connection with the Higher Self comes from knowing we are always loved, guided, and supported by a higher Spirit. This connection to the Source is the bedrock of our lives, and in this realm we do not have to become beautiful, we are that already.

When you begin to connect to the deep Self, you reach a plateau where you face your innermost fears. You may hear that inner voice telling you that you are not worthy. When this neurotic voice is speaking, that part of you that is not connected with your core will feel ugly and less than you truly are. It is the saboteur, diminishing you every chance it gets, in any way possible. This voice may sound like your parent or partner saying you are no good. In fact, you projected this image of yourself onto those people in your life who were not optimally loving.

How you choose to respond to this inner voice is up to you. I suggest that you would be happier if you made the decision to listen to the voice of the Self which loves, accepts, and honors you. It allows you to win and feel good about yourself. It gives you permission to feel beautiful and experience grace. This voice of inner knowing which comes from the depth of your essence never judges you.

I would much rather listen to the voice that loves me and knows I am beautiful, than the one that says I am ugly and unworthy. Listening to the destructive voice wastes my energy and destroys my inner light. The negative voice can be so strong it will never allow me to win or find fulfillment. When I choose the voice that loves me, everything I do—from choosing a hair stylist, to picking a masseuse, or shopping for clothes—will turn out right. I can never make the wrong choice when I love who I am. Daily practice of meditation and reflection enhance this voice so that it becomes loud and clear and drowns out the saboteur.

I feel that grace lives in people who know themselves and love who they are. They know their worth and have learned to build in the necessary self-confidence that reflects their inner light. They are able to show the world the best parts of themselves. Of course, this comes with time, experience, and help from people who like guiding others to become their best. Hopefully, it is incorporated into your spiritual practice and general philosophy about life.

What do you look like when you know who you are? When people have a sense of their worth as well as a deep sense of their personal identity, it is apparent that they have a center which makes everything they do harmonious. It is displayed in how they coordinate their movements, speech, and appearance. It is also reflected in their hairstyle, makeup, and clothing. The negative is also true. If people lack a center, there is something off or disjointed about them, no matter how fashionable they appear or how expensive their image.

I used to dress in soft pastels that showed my gentle nature, but had nothing to say about my level of empowerment, authority, or strength. My friend Sue Bell suggested that I put away the pastels suitable for young girls and start showing my authority, as well as my age. Fearing the responsibility that went with maturity, I resisted her suggestion until I was able to accept the fact that I was hiding from myself. With some inner healing and therapy, I started wearing stronger and deeper colors, and also experienced big shifts in the way I manifested myself in the world.

This came at a time when I had finished my homeopathic studies and was working hard to clear my schooling debts and make a place for myself in the world. This was the time I stopped coloring my hair, and let it go gray. The changes, physical and emotional, were very apparent.

How often have you seen an attractive person who was appropriately dressed for an occasion, but had the wrong haircut, or unsuitable clothes, or wrong makeup? This person was living someone else's ideas about what was suitable. She was not tapping into her own beauty or natural grace. You could sense her desire to be attractive, but on someone else's terms.

Our potential for self-expression changes at each stage of our life. It is inappropriate for a young girl to look thirty or for a mature woman to dress as a teenager. Sometimes, for one reason or another, we become arrested at a certain stage of emotional development, and we act and dress inappropriately, perhaps reflecting our uncertainty about who we are. When we have a strong, resilient relationship with ourselves, and love and honor who we are, we live with and accept the reality of our present physical appearance, and we still maintain a sense of our beauty. There is nothing destructive or dysfunctional showing itself in our appearance. This is a form of self-honesty without brutality and is a statement about expressing our fullest potential. We are doing our best to be our best and this reveals itself in the face we show the world.

I treated a woman for several years who came to see me because she was very unhappy. When I first met her, she looked a good fifteen years older than her actual age because her clothes, hair style, and appearance were very matronly. As she did the necessary inner work and made dramatic changes in her sense of self, her appearance became transformed, on her own accord, and in her own time. She lost weight as she let go of fears and negative thoughts. She longed to wear bright colors and she bought a few new clothes and tried out different ideas to see how she felt and how others responded to her. She was flabbergasted when people she knew were so affirming.

However, this woman had a sister-in-law whose major task in life was putting her down, who naturally did not give her any validation for her new appearance. She eventually came to the conclusion that her sister-in-law's opinion didn't matter and went on with her self-transformation. She had laser eye surgery in order to get rid of the thick glasses she had worn for years, she got a new hair style, and continued increasing her taste in buying clothes. Within a short time, a new woman emerged who was lovely, more confident, and in touch with her inner radiance. She looked like the daughter of the woman I first treated.

Along with her new image came a new level of responsibility for her power and sexuality. She did insist that her husband wake up and start to grow psychologically and spiritually. Both their lives gained verve and vitality. They cultivated joy and well-being in their lives and both looked and felt younger and happier.

If you feel that you already have a harmonious relationship with your Higher Self, you may wish to move on to other sections of this book. If, however, this is new for you, please give this section your attention. It is where the Source of beauty truly lives—within each of us.

LOOKING WITHIN

Looking within is like discovering a clear pool of water. It is still, deep, and serene—it is beauty, joy, and light. If you see anything less than good, you are looking at a reflection of your own dysfunctional ego. When we don't believe we are beautiful, good, loving, or kind, we hold an imposed, prejudicial image of ourselves that is untrue. This image comes from accepting what our family, teachers, and friends imposed on us. In many cases it comes from insufficient love from mothers who may not have had their beauty acknowledged and resented validating it in their daughters. They may have wanted us to conform to a norm that was conventional and safe. Things have changed in the Western world and women are now more empowered. Looking within and finding awareness is now a well-respected path.

We have a Shadow side to our personality, sometimes called accrued negativity. This is meant to be illuminated and eventually released as we purify ourselves and live from an enriched core of being where our invincible connection with Self is located. This awareness is the true path to freedom and beauty. You can choose to let that light shine or you can go on hiding it and conforming to please the world. It is really up to you.

If you are a middle-aged, middle-class woman, there are certain status symbols that define you, just as there are certain symbols that define every age group and social class anywhere in the world. You have the choice to look just like everyone else or you can be yourself and let your beauty shine. If you want more energy, more vitality, and more glow, I suggest it is worth finding your individual sense of beauty. You begin by looking within yourself, not by copying others.

Spiritual people often are found wearing gray, drab clothing with no love for the corporeal expressed in any way. They seem to defy the beauty that is within the human body, which is perhaps the greatest of the gifts we have been given. We are said to be made in the image of God, so how could honoring our physical selves be wrong?

By looking within we have the opportunity to transcend the roles that have been imposed and find what is truly beautiful about ourselves at every stage of our lives. If you have created an image that pleases your partner, your friends, your church, or your mother, it may be time to find an image that really pleases *you*. This may take some experimentation. However, in the end, your image will be a banner of who you are, what you stand for, and how you expect to be addressed. Going within is the first step to connecting with your true Self, where your beauty and grace preside.

This is not about conforming or compromising—it is about being at one with yourself. Take the risk and begin to know yourself from the extraordinary vantage point of love, beauty, and grace. It is what I feel in my heart we are all meant to do at any point in our development.

PRAYER

I think it is inappropriate to tell anyone how to pray. I can make some suggestions that may be useful, but please don't take this as dogma, or as the right or wrong way to engage the Self.

For many years my prayers were like Christmas lists of "give me this and give me that" with the unspoken statement, "I'll do certain things to show my thanks." There is nothing the matter with this form of prayer. It is like a child asking for what he or she wants. I know that for many years of my life it was the only way I knew how to pray. Still other times, especially when there was a crisis, I would desperately ask for deliverance, sometimes just to get through a difficult day. At other times I simply would express my gratitude for the tremendous love that surrounded me, the beauty of the world, and the goodness of people. And, as I matured, I realized how much help and nurturing I had been given.

Now I ask to be shown pathways into my heart and the hearts of those I meet. I realize that Christ consciousness is my goal and that my experiences are not about winning *in* life as much as they are about learning *about* life. This is what helps me purify and heal. As I continue to grow in this awareness of Christ and the love of God I am sure that my prayers will change even more. They will become more like a communion where there are no words, just being with the One within.

I sense that prayer is best done in the morning or evening. After a bad accident recently, I had the opportunity to pray with a group of nuns at Kylemore Abbey in Ireland. The sweetness of their voices praising God brought healing to my soul, and I know that their grace uplifted me and helped me go back to my work and make some important decisions about how I wanted to live my life.

It is important to ask, through prayer, for the healing we need. Even if your prayers are just saying hello to the Presence within you, it is still a connection. You will learn to trust that connection as you continue to call on it to sustain you when times are hard. Prayer keeps us aware that we are not doing it all alone, that there is a Source that guides us and opens doors as we move through life. It reminds us that there is a Plan, even if we can't see it or pretend to understand it.

Prayer is a way to keep the connection open to your inner life. It can take whatever form you are comfortable with — it is not dependent upon any religious practice. All that is asked is that you honor that deep, true part of yourself, in your own way and in your own time.

MEDITATION

There are many forms of meditation that can connect you with your inner Self. They are designed to bring you to the Self gently and comfortably so that you can realize the power and grace of your inner being. The Higher Self works to fulfill the template of your soul's design for your spiritual evolution. Your conscious mind must accept that template and honor the infinite power of creation that works through you. This awareness develops in stages and each stage has its tasks, duties, and rewards just like any level of development.

When we meditate we bring our consciousness away from the world of the senses, duality, and conflicts, and we connect with the One, that essence of being, and the elixir of our soul. When we go within ourselves to the deeper regions of the mind, we calm the mind and slow down our adrenaline-triggered responses to the outer world. This is our time for looking within and releasing tension and pain, finding the light, love, and beauty which is the Self.

In order to meditate you have to create time and space in your life separate from the rest of your waking day. I like to meditate without disruption of the phone or people, where I feel comfortable and can go within. I usually meditate in my bedroom where I can sit against pillows and be comfortable. I like to light a candle and burn incense. Sometimes I will put crystals and pictures of the Buddha, Christ, Indian gods, or the Goddess around an altar. I like to make this time rich in symbolism and as beautiful as possible. I have fresh flowers near me and a mirror so that I can see my inner light reflected in my eyes from time to time.

Meditation is the medicine I need to face my day. When I am writing I have time for lengthy meditation. When I am seeing clients or doing a workshop, meditation becomes more like an exercise to make sure my energy is centered, balanced, and sealed. Either meditation takes me to the same place, which is within, and to the sweetness and beauty of my core.

Meditation is recognized universally as a powerful way to de-stress and revitalize the nerves. For many people it is a true survival mechanism. It is important to meditate regularly. By so doing you will understand where the Source of your power, beauty, strength, and intelligence comes from, and you will become better able to channel this energy into your daily life. It is important to remember that these qualities are coming through you, not from you.

Meditation is the pipeline through which spiritual energy moves in and through your being. Each time you connect with that pipeline you are, in effect, opening yourself to the wisdom, grace, and beauty of the Divine. It actually creates another energy body, called the spirit body, which functions along with the physical body to strengthen and support you.

It's always better to respond to a meditation that you hear. However, you can read the following meditation slowly and try to integrate it into your consciousness. There are also many meditations on tape that you can try.

Meditation for the Self

Sit where you are comfortable and at ease. Meditation works best if you have your seat on a cushion so that your tail bone is slightly higher than your knees. This helps keep the spine straight.

Lengthen your neck by pointing your nose down toward your chest, but keep the crown of your head pointing up toward the sky. This gives you continuous energy flowing from the top of your head to the base of your spine. At this point, you become a transmitter for energy to flow into you from the cosmos, down through your spine and into the earth. As it enters your field it penetrates your seven main energy centers known as the chakras.

Each chakra relates to a color, sound, shape, animal, and planet as well as an archetype of emotional energy. Each center has a system of intelligence that helps you manage your life physically, emotionally, and spiritually. The more you strengthen these centers and balance them, the more you develop spiritually.

Let's go on a journey through the chakras. Take your time and feel your energy shift as you move through these seven major energy vortexes.

The Root Chakra

Let's start this meditation at the base of the spine where the Root Chakra is located and work upward.

This chakra grounds your spirit in life and helps you manifest who you are in the world. Visualize a large red cube big enough to contain your entire pelvis. The planet ruling this chakra is Saturn, which purifies your spirit and gives you a sense of time and patience, as well as an acceptance of reality. A strong Root Chakra focuses your awareness on everyday basics. It makes sure you use your intelligence well to get whatever you need to survive—food, shelter, etc. Without it, you are dependent upon others to look after your everyday needs.

Magnify the size and intensify the color of this red cube. Focus on the qualities of patience, structure, stability, security, and order. Focus on your ability to make your dreams come true. These qualities need only your attention to develop. If you are weak in any area you can develop it with the help of this meditation.

The Sacral Chakra

Now bring your awareness to the area around your navel, known as the Sacral Chakra. Visualize a large orange pyramid which rests on top of the large red cube of the Root Chakra and fills your entire abdomen with its bright orange light. Ruled over by the planet Jupiter, this center controls your emotional responses and the way you physically move. It also is the center for pleasure, creativity, well-being, and abundance. This center has an expansive and warm energy. It is known in Hindi as your own sweet abode.

Expand the size of the orange pyramid and intensify the color. Allow physical beauty, grace of movement, joy, pleasure, sexuality, and prosperity into your energy field.

The Solar Plexus

The Solar Plexus is symbolized by a large yellow globe. Bring your awareness up to your stomach and visualize a strong yellow light that fills your entire upper abdomen and forms a globe of light around your whole body. This is the center of self-worth, confidence, personal power, and freedom of choice. This chakra is ruled over by the planet Mars and the Sun. It is a vital energy center for your sense of personal identity and where you belong in the world. It allows confidence and empowerment to take root here. This is your center for connecting with the world, engaging and controlling your responses to others.

The Heart Chakra

Now bring your awareness up to your chest and to the area of your heart. Visualize a large green crescent moon like a breast plate protecting the vulnerable energy of the heart. It is protecting you from negativity, pain, and attack. The Heart Chakra, like the Solar Plexus, is ruled over by the power and beauty of the Sun as well as the planet Venus.

In your mind's eye, strengthen the green crescent moon by plumping it out and intensifying its color. Know that you are safe to love and be loved and protected from attack from anyone or anything.

The heart itself is a beautiful pink or golden color. It represents the purity and innocence of the human heart and should be protected. Let love be the center of your life and honor your choices for love as you expand the form and intensify the color of this chakra.

The Throat Chakra

Now bring your awareness up to your throat and visualize a beautiful turquoise blue inverted pyramid suspended from the jaw which feeds energy into the mouth, jaw, chin, ears, the neck and throat area. This center is ruled by the planet Mercury, the planet of communication.

The Throat Chakra is the center of truth, communication, will power, and creativity. It acts as a bridge between the feelings of the heart and the thoughts of the mind. If the throat is blocked with unexpressed emotions, this link becomes ineffectual. It is important to open the throat by acknowledging your right to speak your truth and express yourself in the most appropriate and creative ways possible.

Expand the inverted triangle and intensify its turquoise color. Bring light and awareness to this area of your body. Be open to hearing and expressing your truth.

The Brow Chakra

Now bring your awareness up to your forehead and visualize an indigo blue five-pointed star which sends energy down your face toward the tip of your ears, across your eyes and up toward the crown of your head. This center is ruled over by the Moon, the sphere of intuition and inner knowing.

The Brow Chakra controls your ability to discern what and who is for your highest good. It also controls your ability to absorb knowledge and to distill wisdom from your everyday experiences. It controls your imagination and is the center of intuition.

Expand the shape and intensify the color of the blue five-pointed star. Take the star as far back into your head as you can so it can illuminate the far reaches of your mind. Open your mind to your inner knowing.

The Crown Chakra

Now bring your awareness up to the crown of your head and visualize a skull cap of beautiful violet light sitting there. This is the center where you are spiritually connected with the Source. It is not ruled by any planet, since it transcends the zodiac. It is comprised of the qualities of beauty, serenity, and grace. Expand the shape of the skull cap, and intensify the color violet. Allow Spirit to be a part of your life. There is nothing that will sustain you like the love, power, and energy of this center.

You have now shifted your awareness through the rainbow of energy which makes up the human energy system. You can choose from where you want your level of consciousness to flow. You can also help to shift the blocks which stop you from experiencing the flow of energy in your system. The more you do this meditation, the stronger your energy becomes.

Sealing the Chakras with a Cross of Light

Make sure that you seal each chakra before ending this meditation. I do this by visualizing a cross of light within a circle of light, sealing and protecting each delicate energy center. This is a universal symbol of protection which holds the energy of each center intact. I expand this cross of light within a circle of light to include all of me and I crystallize my auric field at the end of each meditation.

When I have balanced my energy I sit quietly and rest in the Oneness of the Source. This is a moment of stillness, being, peace, and beauty. The more you realize this truth of yourself, the more your radiance shines out into the world.

This space is free from pain and tension. It is also a safe place you can retreat to when the world is too demanding. When you begin to be aware of this inner space, you can choose the grace of its gifts to you. This place will sustain you, guide you, and let your talents, gifts, and beauty begin to take expression. It is a place of total trust, goodness, and light.

Take a few moments after meditation to re-enter your present reality. Remember that your senses will be fragile until you re-engage with your ego and the world around you. This meditation can be repeated daily. The more you do it the stronger your energy body becomes and you have more energy for the challenges you face in life. Meditation helps you build reserves of energy that support you during difficult times. It supplies you with the energy you need so you don't appear drained or burned out.

Chapter 2

℘ Connecting with the Archetype of Beauty

We all have models or archetypes to help us live our lives. Each archetype embodies certain quintessential qualities and properties that help us integrate this model of being into our lives. For instance, my archetype of beauty embodies the qualities of serenity, peace, softness, gentility, and grace. I recognize this archetype of beauty by these qualities. Your archetype of beauty can have either a positive or negative impact on you, depending on its function and how you want it to manifest in your life. Your archetype can look like Cinderella, the goddess Minerva, or the Wicked Stepmother. You are the one who chooses the qualities of your archetype.

When you commit your higher consciousness to growth, you strive to create the most beautiful, intelligent, and empowered archetype you can imagine. In so doing you visualize yourself as you would like to be. The next step is to affirm yourself as being worthy of embodying this archetype. It's no good creating the archetype of beauty and then projecting it onto others. You must own your ideals yourself and let them work for you and within you.

Though this will be your intention, visualizing the archetype of beauty is not always done at a conscious level. When you hold on to old and dysfunctional attitudes about your self-worth, you diminish yourself, limit your potential, and create the miasma in which disease and problems occur. You hold in your mind's eye a lesser archetype than your potential to manifest. Wouldn't you rather hold the highest ideal in your mind's eye and let that work as a magnet for your sense of beauty?

Sometimes difficulties show us that we are made of better stuff than we imagined. Have you ever, after a difficult or demanding situation, said to yourself that you were worth more than you received? This suggests that you have a more responsible, empowered, and vital archetype in your mind's eye: i.e., you know you are worth more and deserve better. It will serve you to create a model for your energy which embodies all the qualities of love, intelligence, strength, and beauty you can imagine. A positive archetype enhances the way you see yourself and it assists you in expanding your horizons and opening up to new realms of awareness. When you invoke a loving, intelligent, and beautiful archetype you expand the possibility for your spirit to grow as well. It is as though you can be as big, strong, and enlightened as you are able to imagine yourself to be, and you create this in your mind's eye.

When someone asks you to expand the possibilities and see yourself as beautiful as you can imagine, you may find yourself articulating all the reasons why you couldn't possibly be that way. However, if you are able to expand your possibilities, be careful to keep yourself grounded in the reality of who you are, so that your ego doesn't get out of hand and become harmful or destructive.

This expanded template gives you the chance to examine how you feel about your physical appearance and to listen to your own excuses about why you couldn't possibly enjoy the experience of being beautiful. It is worth noting your resistance to thinking that a transformation is impossible.

Once my good friend Kathy Owen and I had our hair done in new ways and a complete makeup workover for a photo shoot. I was curious to see how I would look with a new image. It was a very professional job and we had a great day and a lot of fun. Kathy's pictures were stunning—and very sexy. When her young son saw them he blushed and said "Mommmm," in the embarrassment typical for adolescents. I knew he had never seen that aspect of his mother before and it surprised him. He wasn't comfortable with that image.

If you were asked to see yourself as beautiful as you could possibly imagine, what would you see in your mind's eye? This is not an easy task. The mind often fails to go into a positive mode and can dwell and stay stuck in the petty details of our appearance. It is easier to dwell on what doesn't work than what potential there is to develop.

This is the critical faculty of the mind responding from your negative model, or archetype, about yourself. It is time to transform your image to fit a new and higher archetype.

The negative aspects of the mind says that a woman your age, your size, in your position, etc., ad nauseum, can't be beautiful. I suggest that it is time to transform the underlying thoughts that you have about yourself and see yourself in a new and positive light. You have the opportunity to have more fun and feel better about yourself if you do. Why not give these exercises a go and see how you feel with a new archetypal image? It gives you the opportunity for eventful growth and inner development by transforming your negative thoughts into positive affirmations. And frankly, it isn't about what you look like but about how you are willing to expand the limits of your narrow vision of yourself that matters. Real development is measured by how far you can push the realms of possibility to more enlightened archetypes.

ARE YOU WILLING TO SEE YOURSELF DIFFERENTLY?

This really is the main question. Are you attached to seeing yourself as you currently are? Are you willing to expand your vision of yourself to include beauty and grace as part of your totality? What stands in your way could be the linchpin to why other things in your life are on hold or don't work.

The optic lens through which you see yourself rather than what you experience is controlling your perception of your beauty. I have seen people transformed during process work where they appear absolutely radiant and stunning. I ask them to look in a mirror and within seconds their face becomes set in the old patterns of self-negation and they lose their glow. This is because they are still attached to seeing themselves in hard, stern, and unloving ways that reflect the ways they were looked at by others. Their optic lens is often punishing and works against themselves.

It takes time to get used to the idea of yourself as beautiful, with inner light shining and radiance. What is asked of you now is the willingness to see yourself differently and in a new perspective. If you are willing to do this, then you can transform your experience of yourself. You won't struggle and the task will be relatively easy.

If you want to struggle and beat yourself up, you can make this a fight with yourself. All the people who programmed you to stop loving and caring about yourself get to be right. If you are willing to open your mind to the idea that you are beautiful, it will open the door to a more loving, joyful, and happy relationship with yourself.

Acknowledging the possibility lets the archetype of beauty grow and take form within you. It also makes you feel that you are beautiful and worthy of your own love and respect. Oddly enough, when you feel this way about yourself, so will others.

In your search for beauty you may want the world to respond to you in a more accommodating way. When you have expectations about how people should see you once you feel beautiful, you begin the process of inflating your ego. Beauty should not be used as a tool to have power over others. A real sense of beauty doesn't need to do this. It graces others and touches the space of beauty within everyone.

You are not responsible for the way the world sees you. Your work is to concentrate on yourself by staying in touch with your feelings and perceptions, and checking them out against a healthy reality factor. Are your perceptions based on the truth of your inner Self or they false delusions that you have invested in for a long time?

If you want to be beautiful so that others will be kinder or more responsive, this exercise will not work. It is not magic nor is it a charm. It merely places your sense of your beauty as separate from the world's acknowledgment. It places beauty within you, within your essence. That is reward enough from the pain of exclusion or dismissal that may have been your experience in the past. When you hold the template of your own beauty, the world has no choice but to respond to you positively. That is how this process functions.

Doing this work, however, does give you the opportunity to feel good about yourself. When you start to love and care for yourself and expand your limited vision of yourself, things change in the world around you. It is not up to you, however, to orchestrate those changes. They happen as a result of the inner shifts in your perception of yourself. So let go of trying to control things and let your beauty find its way into your consciousness. Goodness and fulfillment will follow.

CREATING THE ARCHETYPE OF BEAUTY

In the Greek pantheon of gods and goddesses, Aphrodite was the goddess of love and beauty. Her cult of priestesses and temples existed for over 3,000 years throughout the Mediterranean and especially on the island of Cyprus, which is considered her birth place. The myth of her creation is interesting. In a nutshell, or we should say in a seashell, here is her story.

Cronos was the chief god of Olympus, who had many sons from the goddess of fertility, Hera. Each time a son was born he would kill it. Some children, however, did survive, because of their mother's cunning: Poseidon, the god of the oceans and seas; Apollo, the god of the sun; and Hephaestus, the god of the underworld, valuable metals, and guardian of the souls of the dead.

Hera wanted to save more of her children and gave her next son, Zeus, to a shepherd in Crete to raise. As he grew up, Zeus knew that he was no mortal and eventually went to Olympus to ask for his throne. For years, he battled with his father and many gods joined him: Persephone, Athena, Demeter, Hera, and even Adriadne, Cronos's mistress, accused Cronos of wrongdoing. Hephaestus, Zeus's brother, lent Zeus his art of fire and thunder and Zeus was finally able to defeat Cronos. Cronos asked Zeus to kill him, but instead Zeus castrated him and had the Furies throw his genitals into the sea.

From the mixture of Cronos's sperm and water from the sea, Aphrodite was conceived and born. Others goddesses were more empowered, but she was, by far, the most beautiful. She was worshipped for centuries, first by the inhabitants of Cyprus and then by the Greeks, and finally the Romans who named her Venus. They felt beauty was the essence of life and worshipped it.

Perhaps you have never felt you deserved to be as beautiful as Aphrodite. Certainly, in our world other attributes have been more important for getting ahead in life, and we may have felt it was only the designated few who were chosen to be the beauties.

Each time you pick up a magazine, go to a movie, or watch TV, you are looking at the archetypes of beauty, defined by the advertising media and designers who don't love women's bodies in a realistic way. I would like you to look within yourself to find this goddess. She is there waiting to be brought to life, as in fact all archetypes are waiting to be constellated by our conscious mind. She asks to be welcomed with open arms, and not ridiculed. She may have been lying dormant in you for so long that she is fragile and unsure of herself. Treat her gently, as you keep this work internalized and to yourself until you feel sufficiently confident to share it openly. You shouldn't share your awareness before you feel ready to do so. Bringing our inner goddess into modern times is important. She needs to be appropriately clothed, styled, and made-up to fit into our modern world.

The goddess Aphrodite may have sat in the back of your unconscious mind, prompting you to be more loving and beautiful. Perhaps now is the time to allow her some space in your life. You have been living out everyone else's archetypes of beauty. Perhaps it is time for you to engage with your own internal goddess and model of beauty. Ask her to show you the best of yourself.

When women turn fifty they call on the archetype of the Crone, or the Wise Woman within who guides and nurtures the spirit. She becomes the muse who feeds us on a higher level of creativity. Younger women invoke the archetype of The Mother, The Warrior, The Vamp. Whatever archetypes you have modeled yourself on, it is now time to add a new dimension to your pantheon. Call Aphrodite, goddess of love and beauty, and ask her to show you how she can bring a richer quality to your experience of yourself. Her confidence, radiance, and total assurance can transform how you feel about yourself.

THE GODDESS AS ENERGY

When we speak about mythical characters, be it a goddess or a fairy tale character, we are speaking about an aspect of human consciousness which has universal dimensions. These archetypes are living within us and get acted out in the play of life.

We can consciously choose to identify with them. We can become the Beauty or the Wicked Witch, the Hero or the Damsel in Distress. We also have the ability to transcend these archetypes and re-invent ourselves along the lines of a more empowered and responsible model of beauty, one that is concomitant with our roles in life.

We can identify with different archetypes, such as the Ice Queen, who is cold, frozen, and untouchable, or perhaps we would like to see ourselves as a warmer, more inviting type of beauty. We need only change the image of how we would like to be, and our energy will flow toward that template of creation. What would make you feel happy about who you are? Do you think the Vamp role is worth playing out? Does it hold any promise of intimacy, warmth, love, and fun? Not likely. How do you see beauty being manifested in your fantasy? What are its emotional qualities?

It is important to choose your archetypes carefully, asking yourself what would be for your highest good and greatest joy. Let's consider an archetype that works for you, that helps you get the wholesome attention you want, that gives others the opportunity to respond to you from choice, and not from manipulation.

When we invoke the goddess of beauty, we call on the vast, accumulated knowledge of beauty which women have amassed since the beginning of time. I imagine that cave women used the grease of mastodon fat to rub into their skin to give them added allure. Once in India a woman told me that she washed her face only with water that had been soaked in rose petals and put under the moon every night for a month. She believed it made her beautiful, keeping her young far beyond her real age. She added that the practice had been handed down for generations in her family and was the source of this family's renowned beauty. I tried her method for several months and could see no difference in my complexion. Rather than say that there was something the matter with me, I can conjecture that this woman and her family had constructed a belief that this method worked for them. Invest in any belief and it will work, no matter whether it's cow patties or toad's sperm, expensive face cream, or plastic surgery.

Whether this beauty care is true or not doesn't matter. What is important is that this woman believed it to be true, just like the women who go to Aphrodite's Baths and pat their faces with the water, just like when we invest in expensive creams that offer us the promise of beauty. We believe that it will make us look better, and so it does.

So why not go direct to the Source within yourself and create the quintessential archetype of beauty which will enhance your looks and empower you to be the creator of your own myth? This way you have more control regarding what you choose to buy and use for your beauty care. Wouldn't you rather invest in yourself than project your hope and aspirations into bottles or unguents that are only as good as you believe them to be? It is time to bring beauty into a higher realm of conscious creation and make it less illusion and more real.

Calling the Goddess: Creating a New Model of Beauty

This is a guided meditation taking you through the ancient sanctuary of the goddess Aphrodite, located in Cyprus. There she was worshipped continuously for nearly 3,000 years. Her statue was originally a large black stone, thought to be a meteor, about three feet high. This stone was sanctified by the earliest Bronze Age settlers on this island and thought to have come originally from Asia Minor, where the cult of the Great Mother Cybele originated. The stone signifies the lasting qualities of beauty and love. It wasn't a woman's figure or statue, but a stone that allowed people to invest their own hopes and dreams in love and beauty.

When the Greeks came through Cyprus after their fight with the Trojans, who worshipped the goddess Cybele, they brought with them a beautiful statue of the goddess as we imagine her today. Her statue is lovely, youthful, and wise, and graceful in all her proportions. But in the beginning the stone represented each person's individual belief in beauty and was not a fixed image. It wasn't a prescriptive idea that everyone ascribed toward, but referred to each person's individual beauty. It was as individual as it is for each person who reads this book.

Let us go back into that realm of imagination where we each create our vision of beauty and grace that we wish to experience. Make yourself very comfortable while you read this invocation to the Goddess. Light a candle or burn some incense to help call in Her Divine Essence into your presence. Purify the space you are in by making yourself and your surroundings beautiful and serene.

Now imagine you are about to enter the grounds of the holy Sanctuary of Aphrodite. This temple, which still stands today in the Paphos region of Cyprus, is located on a hill overlooking wheat fields and beyond that, the sea. The sun is shining, there are no clouds, and the color of the sky matches the sea. You come to a gate of the temple and walk through it.

You are walking up sandstone steps graciously spaced apart so that you don't have to strain as you head up toward the temple. The path is lined with fragrant oleander and mimosa. You can smell the orange blossoms, jasmine, and roses. Your senses are awakened by these smells. You walk through a garden of palm trees and eucalyptus which shade the beautiful stone building in front of you and provide shade from the strong sun.

You notice that the walls of the courtyard are adorned with murals depicting the Goddess in her splendor, surrounded by nature. She is, after all, a testament to the beauty in nature as well as in people. Beauty surrounds you everywhere you gaze.

The inner temple is an enormous stone structure which feels alive and vibrant. Through large cedarwood doors, you enter the inner courtyard where a priestess removes your shoes and outer garments. You wash your hands and feet in fresh well water and then are led by a priestess inside the temple itself. The priestess is kind, serene, and gentle, and she smiles at you and takes you by the hand. Nothing is asked of you but silence and reverence.

She gives you a candle as you enter the inner sanctum. It is dark and invitingly cool on your skin. In front of you is a simple altar where you see a large black stone. You approach it and see it is cone-shaped and stands about three feet high. It is the symbol of the power of the Goddess. It contains the wishes, prayers, and projections of women for thousands of years and offers you the sense of the beauty you seek. As you acknowledge the presence of this spirit of love and beauty within yourself, you hear Her voice saying, "Beauty is Yours," as you place your hand on the stone. You are unsure of what you heard and so She repeats the words. You accept that this is your gift from the Goddess and you quietly give thanks and turn to leave.

As you walk around the inner courtyard of the temple, you see the other people who have come to pay respect to Her. They vary greatly in shape, size, color, and age, yet they all revere the Goddess who bestows her unique gifts of beauty to each supplicant. This inspires you to appreciate your gifts as well.

The serenity of this temple overlooking the sea is gentle and makes you happy. You know that the priestesses who honor the Goddess delight in your visit. They smile sweetly at you and nod silently, thanking you for coming. You are now part of the sisterhood that understands the significance of honoring love and beauty. You will be able to know others in the world who honor this Goddess as well.

You leave knowing that this visit to the Goddess has not been a spectacular event — it has simply reinforced your belief in yourself and your worth. You feel very calm. You know that you have been privileged to come close to a universal truth of being which this temple, this stone, and these priestesses represent. They embody the essence of that law of life which you now can bring into your daily reality. You are beauty itself. You can bring this knowledge into your thoughts, your body and appearance, as well as your home and where you work. Beauty is yours.

The Challenge of Beauty

In order to accept this gift from the Goddess, you need to let go of whatever is limiting you in experiencing yourself as beautiful. Your resistance may stem from a complex problem and not have a simple solution. You may also feel confirmed in your belief that beauty is for others and not for you. You will settle for being other things, such as intelligent, well-off, a good mother, or resourceful person. There may be many things that you value about yourself, but you don't consider yourself to be beautiful.

What would it take for you to feel that you are beautiful? Does it take a man or woman telling you that you are beautiful? Does it need to come from your father or your mother? If they told you so, would you believe them?

We play so many games hiding our awareness of our beauty. We feel that beauty is for the young, the slender, the white, the rich, other people, but not for us. Are you willing to live with this limitation and hide behind this projection?

I have seen women who were not beautiful by any stretch of the imagination transform a room with their presence. They felt beautiful and their radiance captivated everyone. Of course, there were the usual critics who tried to pull these women apart by looking for things to criticize, but they couldn't put their finger on the elusive quality of their beauty. These women would carry their beauty to their graves. You can't put an age limit on it and narrow it down to its components such as hair, makeup, or clothing. It is an inner quality.

Cultivating beauty is possible for everyone. No one can give you this awareness, you have to want to make it a part of yourself. You have to feel that you are worthy of it and have every right to feel beautiful. This is the essence of your magic, your grace, and your sense of Self.

Don't expect validation from a world that only sees beauty as wearing the right brand of sunglasses or designer labels. No, the world doesn't validate this inner quality. It can't even see it most of the time. You need to create the feeling and delight in its radiance and bathe in your essence of self daily until it is strongly re-enforced within you.

EXAMINE YOUR ATTITUDES ABOUT BEAUTY

Look at your attitude about your own beauty. Your negativity will amaze you if you criticize yourself constantly. At the end of the day you will be left feeling ugly, or not good enough. You can see that your own attitude is preventing you from experiencing yourself as beautiful. How dreary, when you have been working so hard at self-development, to get bogged down with this negative attitude which you probably think can't be altered.

I recently read an interview with a very beautiful woman who reported how much she disliked herself. Her modesty did not become her, and in fact I suspected she suffered from a serious neurosis. What a shame to think that we are not good enough. What is the model of perfection we hold ourselves against and what is enough? Why should our natural right to beauty be so hard to attain? Why do we punish ourselves this way?

INTERNALIZING APHRODITE

We can internalize any archetype into our consciousness—we can become what we wish to be. When we take Aphrodite within us, she manifests her beauty in our mind's eye. We can ask her to help us develop a healthy sense of our own beauty.

We can bring her qualities of serenity, grace, and loveliness into our hearts and minds, and integrate them within us. We can give ourselves permission to be soft, open, and radiant whenever we choose. Her qualities soften our voice, as we stop punishing ourselves. We may even consider changing our way of berating ourselves and may even smile at ourselves in the mirror from time to time.

How does self-acceptance come about? We have to live love and beauty. It becomes manifested in the loving and tender gestures we make toward others; it shows when we give ourselves permission to take a day off to rest and treat ourselves to a massage or an ice cream. It may include working out at the gym, going for a swim, planning a wonderful holiday with a friend. There are so many ways to be good to yourself. You can begin to love the person you are and let your beauty be visible in small, unobtrusive ways. You can begin by not being as strict about what you do. You can temporarily stop the pushing and striving and give yourself a rest. Beauty shines best when we are rested and peaceful.

Take a look at the other ideas in this book to see if something attracts you to enhance your beauty. There is no point doing something you don't want to do. Enjoy yourself. It is part of finding your beauty.

Do What Makes Your Heart Sing

The Goddess comes to life in us when we are happy and fulfilled. This is the best way we embody her archetype. She sings and smiles through us when we love ourselves and the people around us.

There are many people who haven't explored what makes them happy. When I ask them that question, they are surprised. Most people believe that they have to do what they are doing, and that they essentially have no choice to change.

I have discovered it takes very little to make people happy. Actually, it is the simplest things that give us the most pleasure. I have also been surprised to find how little time people devote to the things that give them pleasure, compared to the time they devote to the things that leave them frustrated and upset.

Do we have to spend our lives suffering? The question is worthy of consideration. If you really believe that you have to suffer in order to please God or your family, then everything in your life will make you suffer. I am suggesting that if something is chronically draining your resources and your energy, it might do you good to examine it. What motivates you to keep on doing the very thing that hurts you? Wouldn't you rather risk doing something else that gives you joy, even if you had to change some things in your life to do so? When people do things they enjoy, their beauty radiates. We see this on the faces of people who love their lives and what they do.

What Especially Makes Your Heart Sing?

Doing what makes your heart sing releases endorphins from your brain into your bloodstream and makes your whole body relax and feel good. Struggle, especially repeated struggle, wears people down and weakens their immune system. When we give ourselves even fleeting moments of pleasure, we boost our defenses against disease and expand our energy field with joy and vitality.

There are times when people are committed to seeing an important or challenging matter through, and their resources and energy are completely absorbed in meeting this situation. They develop strength of character and will power from doing this and there is a deep level of commitment and responsibility in these people. These people are beautiful because they show us that service and surrender are also aspects of beauty. This comes from the soul.

Drawing the line between doing something that is draining and miserable and something you are committed to seeing through is really up to you. No one can tell you what to do with your life. It is up to you to decide if what you are doing is worth it or not. If it is what you truly want, then your heart will sing and your beauty will shine no matter how little sleep you get.

I know that when people are engaged in a difficult task they can do well to take time out to smell the roses and do the simple things in life which bring pleasure. A good friend of mine is nursing her sick husband. She sings, gardens, and speaks to her friends and support network regularly. Her beauty seems to grow every time I see her. Her radiance is apparent to everyone because she does her task with love, commitment, and courage. She has accepted her task with grace and gives her all to it. She often goes without sleep for nights on end, staying awake to be with her husband. She has been an inspirational teacher and friend to me, showing me how love and beauty can flourish in difficult circumstances. Her soul is radiantly visible.

What are you willing to do to bring more joy into your life?

Can you make a list of the things you really love doing? See how many are possible for you. When you have done this, see how many can be implemented now.

Ask yourself, "What do I want to do now that will give me joy and make my heart sing?" It may be as simple as fixing a cup of tea or going for a walk. Pleasure is not complex. When you let these experiences add up throughout the day, they make for a happy face and warm demeanor. It is surprising how much a little pleasure can do to turn a dull or ordinary day into something unique.

The more pleasure you are willing to let into your life the more beautiful you will be. Those frown and worry lines will begin to disappear and your complexion will radiate light. We think that muscles sag because of gravity. More correctly, the gravity of our life makes muscles sag. It is time to lighten up and find some small, simple pleasures that help recharge your vitality.

Many years ago in Brussels I was walking down the fashionable Avenue Louise and saw a lady wearing what appeared to be a very expensive Chanel suit, shoes, and handbag. She was dripping diamonds from her hands, ears, and throat. Her makeup and hair style were impeccable, but her face was sour and her shoulders slumped. All the money in the world couldn't buy her beauty. The choice for health, happiness, and well-being is ours, and no amount of money can make that happen. It is an inner quality reflected outward to the world. We must choose radiance from within. When we do, we nurture the goddess within ourselves and give our light the opportunity to shine.

Find the light of your Higher Self, honor the goddess of love and beauty within by seeing what genuinely makes you smile. Affirm your worth and visualize how you would like to see yourself. This is the basic foundation for all beauty.

Chapter 3

❧Affirming Your Worth

Without a basic belief in yourself, any attempt to feel beautiful will fail. If you have spent a lifetime thinking you were less than beautiful, affirmations can help you re-program your conscious. They require vigilance every time you allow yourself to think old, negative thoughts, but you can make them fun by singing them in the shower, or reciting them into a tape recorder and saying them as you exercise. You can write them down and place them around your home and where you work. I place them on my telephone, my mirrors, and the wall next to my bed so I can say them to myself when I wake up and go to bed.

Affirmations remind us that we can have a healthier attitude about ourselves. They can help increase your energy, bringing love, beauty, abundance, and health into your life. They work by keeping the mind fixed on an idea which, with time and focus, penetrates the subconscious, where transformation takes place. They can eradicate our negative ideas and give us hope for a better future.

Affirmations help re-balance our energy field. They work on

the principle that we are responsible for the quality of our experiences, and that by thinking positive thoughts about ourselves we can transform ourselves and our experiences. When we think positively, like magnets, we attract positive situations and people that bring us the experiences we need for our healing and development. This is how we change and heal.

Affirmations allow us to see our negative side, and replace stale and worn-out attitudes with positive thought forms. Wouldn't you rather reinforce a belief that life is good? When we do so, we have a chance to purify our spirit and strengthen our mind. Our affirmations open us to a new realm of possibilities. They are positive statements of intent to the Universe.

In my workshops I sometimes show participants how a pendulum works. I hold it over the Solar Plexus and ask the participant to recite the following affirmation: "I am beautiful and everyone loves me." The energy that this generates within the person's electromagnetic field produces a swing of the pendulum in a positive direction. The more vigorously she repeats it, the stronger the pendulum swings.

I then ask the person to say, "I am ugly and no one loves me." The energy that this generates shifts the pendulum and makes it turn in the other direction or makes it stop altogether. This exercise illustrates how strong your negative and positive thoughts are and how they influence your life force and energy field.

SPECIAL AFFIRMATIONS

It often is productive to repeat affirmations while you are in the shower, driving, or doing other tasks that don't require full attention. They are best done using a mirror — the most confrontational, direct way for you to challenge your attitudes is to look yourself in the eye. You can actually see yourself change as you repeat positive statements.

If you are going to let your obsessions about yourself stop you from experiencing your own beauty, you are shortchanging yourself. The mirror work gives you an opportunity to hear your own critical voice. Just think how easy it is for others to criticize you when you have shown them the way. Other people mirror our self-regard.

Exercises

Begin by standing in front of the mirror and telling yourself that you are beautiful. Smile at yourself, delight in yourself, and be aware that this is how you would like to be seen. Do this until you feel in your body that you are telling the truth about yourself. Accept yourself as you are, with love. Stay there for as long as it takes to remove the pain and resentment from your eyes. Make some gestures of reconciliation and love while looking in the mirror and repeating the affirmation. See what happens. You may find how much you actually love and care for yourself.

You can practice this every time you pass a mirror. Give yourself a look that says that you are lovely, someone you'd like to know and enjoy. Blow yourself a kiss from time to time. Love what you see, accept yourself, and value this person that is you.

The next step is to stand in front of a full-length mirror without your clothes on. Try not to get caught up with what you dislike about your body. Look at yourself and say you accept and love yourself just the way you are. Tell yourself that you are beautiful. Acknowledge that your body has done a wonderful job supporting you in the best way it could for all these years. Your body has worked hard for you. It deserves care, rest, exercise, good food that nourishes you, and plenty of water, air, and pleasure. How you decide to integrate these things into your life is up to you. When you learn to give yourself exactly what you need, you will be content and happy with yourself just as you are.

Whenever you are physically moving your body is another good time to affirm yourself. You can swim your affirmations, do them whenever you are repeating a movement at the gym, or when you are out walking or jogging. We all need some form of exercise and this is an excellent time to do affirmations. It will make your task more enjoyable and give you more energy. Try it and see.

These are ways that you can energize your body at the same time that you feed the subconscious mind where your attitudes are stored. Take time to let these affirmations work. You may need to repeat them many times for several weeks. When you feel they are integrated into your being, stop repeating them and let them work for you.

CREATING AFFIRMATIONS WHICH SERVE YOUR SELF-WORTH

We have acknowledged that there is no beauty, and for that matter no healing, without a sense of worth. The implications of this are deep and profound. I ask people in workshops what they think they have to do to be worthy of love, beauty, and healing. The answers are as varied as the people.

In truth, there is nothing you have to do to be worthy of love or beauty. It goes with the territory of being human. People who do exaggerated spiritual practices, lengthy pujas, endless hours of purification, long fasting diets, and endless workshops to develop their worth miss the point. You already have it. Just make that internal connection to it and it is yours. Those other things are done to raise energy vibrations, to bring awareness and release to the body, and to purify the spirit. They do not in any way bring you self-worth. You have to know within yourself that you are worthy simply because you exist.

From this point we can look at some affirmations which help you enhance your worth. When you think about the things you want in life, ask yourself if you are worthy of them. Hopefully the answer is yes. Whether you get them, how you handle them once you have them, what happens to your development during this time, are different issues altogether. But, yes, we are all worthy of the things we say we want.

Many years ago I realized that people spent so much money on beauty products and treatments because they were searching for their self-worth through looking and feeling good. There is nothing the matter with wanting to look or feel good. It is a mistake, however, to think that self-worth comes attached to your physical appearance.

We all have moments, even long periods of time, when we may feel unloved or not cared for. To brood over these times feeds our narcissism, the belief that we deserve to be special. This is exactly the time when we need to do inner work and find our strength and resources. These are the times we have to find love for ourselves and learn to nurture the person inside who is lonely and fragile. We can become our own inner parents and resolve our sense of loss and abandonment through the awareness of our worth. This is real healing.

If we cling to the belief that others are responsible for our welfare and happiness, we can turn sour and dislike the people who are doing the best they can to support us, love us, and be our friends. As adults, no one is responsible for us. We alone are responsible for the quality of our experiences.

When we know that we are worthy, we may look at ourselves and others in a different light and understand our own limitations. This exercise is not designed to feed anyone's rampant narcissism about what she feels she deserves. Taking responsibility begins now. You have the power within you to transform your life and it starts here and now. So let go of the past, acknowledge your feelings, and move on to a place where you feel positive about yourself and willing to make your life work.

The following affirmations have been created for you. You can use these or you can make up your own. Do what is comfortable for you and find affirmations you feel happy using. You can repeat them as often as you like. Stop saying them when you feel that the affirmation has been integrated into your subconscious mind. You will experience your negativity gradually fading away as you replace it with more positive and wholesome thoughts about yourself.

I love myself.

I honor my worth.

Life supports me in being the best that I can be.

Everything I do expresses my sense of self-worth and love.

I do my best in all circumstances to love myself.

When things appear challenging I look within to the place of love and light. I find the highest point of love within me.

I know that I am always worthy of love, kindness, and respect.

I find my worth in everything I do.

Life is affirming me each day in every way.

I deserve the best and I know the best will come to me.

The more I honor my worth the more I feel worthy to have and enjoy the good things in life.

My nature is divine. It is eternal, loving, wise, intelligent, and beautiful.

Beauty is mine now.

I am open to being, feeling, and looking the best I can.

I accept myself exactly as I am. I love myself and I honor my worth.

I am worth my weight in gold, diamonds, and rubies.

I am worth all that I feel is good, wholesome, and loving.

Love is the center of my life.

I create health, wholeness, and beauty for myself.

I bask in the serenity of beauty and love.

I know that I am loved, protected, and guided at all times.

I tap into my natural resources of love, freedom, and beauty.

I accept that beauty is a natural part of who I am.

Beauty expresses itself through me in the way I move, think, and do things in life.

Beauty is the expression of who I am.

I am beautiful!

No matter what my age, size, shape, or skin color, no matter what afflictions I have, my beauty is there to be experienced and expressed.

I love who I am and my beauty is an expression of me.

I give thanks for the beauty that is in me and surrounds me.

Life is beautiful.

I am a radiant, conscious, and loving person.

I see love, beauty, and grace when I see myself.

Beauty surrounds me and nurtures my soul.

Who I am is loveliness, beauty, and grace.

I appreciate the power of beauty and love to transform my life.

Chapter 4

✌Visualizing Your Beauty

Visualization is a technique used by many therapies for a variety of needs: for people who are ill; or for whenever the mind is arrested in a fixed or a rigid pattern where existing reality does not support health, healing, or creativity; or when the mind needs a gentle stretch to spur on its power and creativity.

Most of us have lost the wonderful gift of imagination. It disappeared around the time we started school and if it lingered any longer, we were persuaded to stop daydreaming. We are going to use the imagination as a tool for assisting our inner work of establishing a healthy context for beauty. As with all skills, the imagination needs to be exercised to stay functional and serve its purpose, which in our adult lives helps us see the dreams we want in life. Our imagination has the power to create this reality and bring us joy, happiness, and prosperity.

We have the capacity to imagine a job we like or the kind of person we would choose for a mate, or a home we'd like to live in. Imagination is a gift from God. With it we can create our reality as we would like it to be. Let's use it to create a picture of ourselves looking beautiful and feeling radiant.

CREATING A SENSE OF OUR OWN BEAUTY

We will harness our imagination to expand our sense of beauty. Unlike affirmations, visualization needs to be done only a few times—once, twice, at the most. It can, however, take much longer to imagine what you really want.

Once the picture is created in your mind's eye it can be played back to remind you what you asked for. It acts as a template of creation to manifest what your heart desires. Think carefully about how you would like to see yourself. Find the qualities that best express your beauty and your sense of Self.

As an example of how visualization works, I tell a story how I wanted to live in a lovely place in the country and visualized a cottage surrounded by roses. That was all that I could see. Within days a house came on the market in the country. It had roses all around the house, along with many other features I could never have imagined, including a beautiful conservatory where I write, looking out at an old and beautiful garden, and hills in the distance.

We can visualize our bodies the way we wish them to be, and with continued work we form the template that our body can mold itself into. We can see our complexions smooth and youthful. We can see our carriage and movements graceful and coordinated. If you have any physical problems, you can see them changing form. You can see yourself any way you want. Invest that image with energy and you have the makings of fulfillment.

I recently heard a story about a young man who after a serious car accident was faced with having his foot amputated. He worked with a healer, visualizing himself walking with both feet in good condition. He did this several times daily and within weeks was able to regain the use of his foot. You may think it ridiculous that imagination could do this. Yet this story and others appear in our medical journals daily. The mind creates the template that reality molds itself into.

Another story comes to mind of two basketball teams in training. The first team was asked to visualize making perfect shots. They sat in chairs for several hours every day for a week doing this mental exercise. The second team practiced on the court shooting baskets for a week. At the end of the week the two teams met. The team that had visualized the baskets scored three times higher than the team that had practiced. These days this technique, called the Inner Game, is utilized by coaches. Let's use it to access our inner beauty.

CREATING THE PERFECT ENERGY FIELD FOR YOURSELF

Start visualizing a resourceful and healthy energy field. See yourself active, see yourself from about four feet away in your mind's eye. Imagine your body strong and healthy. It supports you and is full of energy and vitality. See the features you like enhanced and the features you don't like more in harmony with the rest of your body.

You may have short legs, flat or too large breasts, large hips— whatever you consider defects, use your mind's eye to diminish it. See yourself in a hologram where you like the image that you see. This is you as you would like to be from an energetic and physical point of view.

See yourself smiling, even laughing. See yourself confident, content, and fulfilled. This is the you that you would like to become. See your beauty shining in your eyes and in your smile. You know how lovely you can be when you are really happy. Give that to yourself now.

Now come up close to your hologram and see your face, the face you always wanted to have, lovely, glowing with beauty, and very alive. See yourself smiling and laughing and your complexion clear and smooth. Your eyes are alive and there are no sagging, pulled down lines anywhere on your face. Your teeth look strong and healthy and your neck is strong and firm.

Hold this image even if it doesn't match your current reality. Affirm this vision by saying you like what you see. Embrace this image. Give it your approval. Sharpen the focus so that you see the small details of your face. Put the image you desire into this visualization.

Use your imagination to smooth away the things you don't like. You may have wrinkles you would like to see diminished, or bags and puffiness around your eyes or mouth. You may have unwanted facial hair you want removed, or growths or discolorations that are not attractive. Use your imagination to remove anything about your face that does not appeal to you. See it in a gracious and loving way. Accept it and cherish it. This is the face you show the world.

You can shorten your nose, build up your chin, straighten your teeth. With your mind's eye you can hold your face in the image you like. This is internal plastic surgery and it works at a very deep level to help you transform your sense of yourself. The power of creation is in your imagination and it is working for you.

During the day you can hold this picture of your energy field, your face, and physical body in front of you. Don't dwell on it but remember what you want to see. It is all part of your finding your sense of beauty and using the power of your mind to achieve your desire.

Visualizing Yourself As You Would Like to Feel

The essence of this work is how you re-invent yourself so that you look and feel the way that suits you. Begin to imagine the delight, joy, and happiness to go along with the energy, body, and face you want. Start by feeling this way now.

Imagine what it feels like to be at ease with yourself and your life. You still have the problems you have now, but your attitude to those problems are different. You slow down a bit and start to smell the roses more. Life feels less tense and more relaxing.

You may want to see yourself doing something that would embody these qualities. You might imagine yourself walking in the country, sailing on a boat, skiing down a mountain, sitting on a comfortable sofa, feet up, and watching a good film. Whatever image of yourself is at ease and happy, put into your mind's eye now.

You can see yourself sleeping in and the clock saying its nearly noon, or walking around in your nightgown eating toast, reading the paper, or watching TV. What would be symbolic of ease for you? Can you say yes to this image? Let it seep into your consciousness so that you can accept the sense of ease as a natural part of your life.

Now let's imagine being creative. This can take any form you would enjoy: playing a musical instrument, singing with friends, painting, embroidering, making an outfit for yourself, gardening, or cooking a good meal for your friends and family. See yourself doing something you really like and experience the feelings of happiness. Hold that vision and say yes to it. Allow creativity into your life, and know you deserve to give yourself the time to do the things you like.

Now let's imagine time for recreation: swimming, dancing, yoga, climbing mountains, or simply walking in the country. You could be riding a bike or skiing. See yourself moving in some way that feels good to you. You are delighted with the way your body feels after you have done this.

Now say yes to moving in a way that stimulates your body to do whatever it needs to stay healthy and support you. Allow yourself to feel alive. Allow physical well-being to be a part of your experience.

Now let's imagine a deeper sense of beauty. See yourself dressed for a special event—a wedding, celebration, anniversary, or birthday. See yourself in a lovely dress that shows off your grace and elegance. See yourself wearing the right accessories that would make this outfit perfect. The right shoes, jewelry—anything you need so that you look and feel absolutely perfect.

Now see your hair and face. Your hair is in a style that suits you perfectly. See your smiling face, perfectly made up to show off your best features. You look absolutely glowing and radiant. Notice the people around you are smiling and happy to be sharing this moment with you. Now hold this image of yourself and say yes to it. Say that you are willing to let this picture of yourself manifest into reality. Remember the feeling, remember what you look like. When this materializes, remember that you embodied the power to create this for yourself.

If there is any other area of your life you wish to visualize, take the time to create it the way you want it to be. You may want to see yourself with abundance, friends, and good health. Use your creative powers to manifest a life and physical appearance that give you pleasure and happiness.

Part II

Living Beauty:
Loving and Nourishing
the Body

Chapter 5

℘ Relaxing for Life

Once we have created the foundation for honoring our inner beauty, the next step is to look after and care for ourselves. We nourish the physical body so that it can function optimally and serve our expanded inner consciousness. Caring for the outside, which is the external manifestation of ourselves, is as important as centering on the inside.

Today, people are obsessed with how well or poorly their bodies function. Everywhere I go people are talking about their health and what they are taking to make themselves feel well. Yet, for all the preoccupation, there seems to be little regard for the way the body operates as an energetic unit.

Without an awareness of energy, we are left with a fragmented understanding of ourselves. We examine and treat each aspect of ourselves as separate units. We fail to see that we are a whole, a totality of energy in which every part of the body reflects a state of well-being or disease. Accepting ourselves as an energetic unit means that we accept the mind/body/spirit as a continuum of energy in which each of these three components is synergistically related to the other two.

If we see ourselves as machines that need to be fueled, rested from time to time, and repaired when something breaks down, we may treat ourselves ruthlessly and fail to tap into the beauty, joy, and grace available to us. When we see ourselves as energy, we respect the life force that moves in and through us and which can heal and transform us. We honor the temple that is the vessel to our energy by giving it food that feeds the soul and the body, medicine that works along energetic principles, and exercise that molds the body into a support unit for our daily tasks.

The body has an intelligence far beyond our conscious mind. If we tune in and listen, we can learn our history, feel our inheritance, experience and release our sorrows, transmute our fears, and our expand our hopes. The body is the living presence of Spirit. Giving it less than the best condemns us to disregard who we truly are.

THE IMPORTANCE OF RELAXATION

In considering the care of the body, we begin with relaxation. So many of our problems would vanish if we could simply find peace of mind. Relaxation techniques release the stress and strain from our body and ease our minds, freeing both to function at their best.

We live in stressful times. Most of us have highly demanding lifestyles with pressure to perform at work, financial ups and downs, and the juggling act of too many responsibilities and activities. Many of us are pushing our bodies to their limits or beyond. We are constantly in a rush, running on forced levels of adrenaline, which wears out our nerves and immune systems. We only rest when we hit the crash-and-burn point and collapse. To live your life in this cycle of running and collapsing is abusive to your body, an abuse similar to the yo-yo syndrome of starving and gorging yourself. Your body will eventually break down, no amount of will can sustain it at this pace. This fast pace will burn out your energy and destroy your beauty.

Are you willing to look at how you treat yourself and the demands you make on yourself? It may be a matter of life and death for you to examine your level of intense activity and ask what purpose it serves. Do you really need to push that fast and that hard? If you do choose to continue at this pace, are you prepared to take the time to rest and regenerate? How often do you give yourself the chance to be still and let healing occur?

It's a lot harder to reverse the effects of damage than prevent it. Making changes before you reach the breaking point is a way to honor your Self. Giving the body the pleasure, rest, and relaxation on which it thrives will enable it to handle times of stress and pressure.

If you want to play for high stakes, you have to learn to manage your energy. For people who are fixated on activity, relaxation can be seriously hard work. Few people have the ability or give themselves permission to stop "doing" for any length of time and simply relax. You have to learn how to give yourself permission to discover what is relaxing for you. It can take many forms. What one person sees as relaxation may be another person's idea of stress. Some people, to others' disbelief, find cleaning their house or sorting out a closet very relaxing. Others may jog five miles a day. Others may enjoy painting or reading.

The rest of this chapter is devoted to a discussion of techniques which I have found useful as ways of slowing down and relaxing. I use some on a daily basis and others when I am busy teaching and working with people. They always bring me back to myself, ease me back to pleasure, and restore my peace of mind and sense of well-being.

While the techniques come from a variety of disciplines, they all involve the ability to turn the mind off momentarily and to bring ease and release tension in a highly stressed system.

BREATHING FOR LIFE

Nothing will ease and de-stress the body and mind faster than taking a few good breaths. When people are under stress, in crisis, or traumatized, their breathing tends to slow down and become shallow and weak. Breathing in this way reduces the supply of oxygen to the body's cells. The heart, lungs, and brain don't work as well. Lactic acid builds up in the muscles, making us feel tired and sluggish. In cases of panic or extreme anxiety, breathing becomes too rapid, and hardly any oxygen is released into the bloodstream or brain.

Proper breathing releases the right amount of vital oxygen into the blood and soothes the nerves. Most people need to work their lungs to keep their bodies oxygenated. If you are troubled or worried, take a few minutes off simply to focus on inhaling and exhaling. This can help restore your equilibrium and bring you back to awareness of yourself. Respiration is, after all, a primary function of the body. To stay clear, healthy, and relaxed, it is important that you use your breath consciously.

Techniques which work with the breath, such as yoga and bioenergetics, are useful. In yoga, the breath is controlled to regulate the sympathetic nervous system and reduce the flow of adrenaline in the body. Bioenergetics, on the other hand, engages the breath to release suppressed emotions locked into the musculature of the body. It stimulates the flow of adrenaline to awaken these deep feelings which then surface in the conscious mind, thus finding an outlet for expression.

Singing is marvelous for keeping the breath open. It releases the blocked energy accumulated in your chest and lungs, simultaneously energizing and relaxing you, and lifting your spirits. It can help increase your capacity for joy as well.

Any physical activity is an opportunity to work with your breath. Try to coordinate your breathing with your movements. When you breathe consciously, it creates harmony and gives you a sense of energy flowing through you. Breath is life.

Here are some exercises to help you become aware of your breathing.

Conscious Breathing Exercises

Whenever I feel pressured by stress, I use a technique known as conscious connected breathing, which uses stillness and concentration. I have found it effective for dealing with emotional blocks as well as strengthening my life force and helping me relax. Through this form of breathing, I learned the power of the breath to restore a sense of well-being instantly.

The first technique requires nothing more than easy, conscious breathing for a few minutes. In a crisis or whenever I experience fear or shock, if I turn my awareness to my breathing for a few minutes, I recall who I am and let go of my fears. My defenses melt, and my body once again feels relaxed and at ease.

The breath is life's natural energy cleanser and can rebalance us quickly, yet we so often forget to do it. Begin by turning your attention to your breathing and breathe naturally. Does your breath come easily or are you aware that your breathing is tight and forced? Take a few moments at different times during the day to focus on your breathing. At first, you may need to remind yourself to do this, but eventually it becomes habit.

When you have time, sit in a chair or lie down for ten to fifteen minutes and breathe deeply, not pausing between breaths. You should be breathing rhythmically and effortlessly. You need do nothing but concentrate on your breathing. If time and place allows, you can light a candle or burn incense. You might also rub some soothing aromatic oils on your forehead and temples.

For the next technique, you need a snorkel. I lie down in my bathtub with my head underwater, and breathe rhythmically for about five minutes. This energizes my body by releasing deeply held tension. If you don't want to get your hair wet, use a close-fitting bathing cap.

When I am on holiday at the sea or by a lake, I lie face down in the water and float, breathing through a snorkel and letting the water roll over me for as long as I can, several times a day. It is deeply relaxing and very soothing to the spirit. Floating in clear water, simply breathing in and out, puts me into my most relaxed state. It is a state of bliss, reminiscent of being back in the womb.

Rest

Rest only comes when you stop pushing and striving, and let down your defensive stance. It gives you the opportunity to regain a sense of ease and pleasure. Rest will balance you, allowing you to recharge and unwind. It is essential for a healthy life.

Nothing ages people faster than the stress of the fast lane, bolting ahead, burning adrenaline, and seeking constant stimulation.

In our culture, we are inundated by visual and auditory stimulation, and have become addicted to the point that silence and stillness frighten us. We live with the radio or television on constantly. Today people fear solitude and silence, the bliss that mystics have sought through the ages. We put so much emphasis on moving forward that people have difficulty simply being still.

The body requires a balance between activity and stimulation on the one hand and tranquillity and rest on the other. Today we ignore the rest and tranquillity half of the equation. As a result, immune system breakdown and diseases are virtually epidemic. Before you reach the breaking point, why not pay attention to your body's signals, such as the dark rings under your eyes or frazzled nerves, that you need more rest?

Rest helps you develop a sense of beauty. A friend once told me that all the great beauties of the last century believed they required one day a week in bed resting. While tending to our beauty may not be part our profession, it is part of our life's work.

When you are worn out from overexertion, beauty doesn't have a chance to thrive or be fulfilled. The body is devoting all of its energy to trying to keep up with the demands created by your ambitions and strivings. Beauty is not born from tension and drive.

Simply by resting more, you can increase your sense of well-being and regain some of your lost beauty. Rest can mean going to bed earlier during your work week and sleeping in on your days off. These are short-term ways you can rest. It's important also to give yourself longer periods of rest such as extended weekends and holidays when you can rest more fully.

You may find that you need a break every few months from the routines of your life. Beautiful places reinforce the idea that you don't need to strive so hard to get the things you want in life.

When you breathe in the healing spirit of nature, you remind yourself that life was meant to be enjoyed, and that it's important to take time to smell the roses.

Saying no to pressures and people that sap your vitality may help you give yourself the rest you need. I have observed that people habitually in a state of stress have trouble defining their boundaries and get burned out by doing too much to prove their worth. Often, they don't stop until they are forced to do so when their immune system becomes depleted.

Accidents and less than optimal work are signals that rest is overdue. People who are tired make errors in judgment and mistakes. Companies are now recognizing the benefits of implementing periods of rest and relaxation for workers. The practice increases productivity and incentive, and keeps people recharged and happier.

If your life has pressures, and whose doesn't, and you don't have a program of rest and recuperation that suits you, it's time to implement one. In many countries, business shuts down in the middle of the day to give people an opportunity to relax and enjoy lunch and rest afterward. They then are refreshed, able to tackle their afternoon's work easily. In our society, we usually bolt down our food, often while working at our desks.

Consider what amount of time you can devote each day to rest—even small breaks during the day make a difference. Can you give yourself moments of silence, away from machines, outside in the fresh air and sunlight? Even taking a walk around the block goes a long way toward refreshing your body and giving you a boost for the rest of the day. You will feel better, and it will renew your sense of well-being and beauty. Build rest into your life and you will give yourself more quality time for enjoying the good things in life. And remember, it is very hard to feel beautiful when you are exhausted.

SLEEP

A doctor once told me that the hours you sleep before midnight are for your beauty, whereas the hours after midnight are for your body. With this in mind, you might want to consider a fuller night's sleep. It can resuscitate you, giving you the energy you need to meet the challenges of your life. You will look and feel better for doing it.

Periods of hibernation are also a part of all life cycles. Nature uses the fallow time of winter to nurture life energy that will emerge again in the spring. The body's sleep cycle is essential to maintaining healthy balance in the human energy system. We use sleep to refresh and renew all of our body's needs. It is said we heal in sleep. During sleep, the blood is cleansed, the kidneys, which are the seat of life force, rest and rejuvenate. Sleep restores the fluidity of the lymph, which helps eliminate toxins. It also re-establishes the osmotic pressure of the cells and reactivates their life energy. Sleep enables the cycles of the body to rebalance themselves. When sleep is dysfunctional, all the body's cycles are thrown off.

A healthy sleep cycle is essential for emotional and psychological well-being. In sleep, we process stress and conflict. It is nature's psychic clearinghouse for mental and emotional overload. Sleep opens the door to the unconscious mind, which speaks to us through our dreams, guiding us toward a healthy future. We need to be willing to listen to our own internal truths disguised as metaphors, symbols, and images in our dream content.

With its effect on all levels of being, sleep is a natural beauty aid. Take some time off to restore yourself in sleep and watch the sparkle return to your eyes and the glow of your skin.

If your sleep cycle is disturbed in some way, try to restore balance through natural methods. Sleeping pills will not give you the deep sleep cycles you need in order to feel refreshed. You actually feel worse from taking these drugs, which are also addictive and cause dependency problems.

Excellent homeopathic remedies and herbal tinctures are available in health food stores and other outlets. I recommend the following homeopathic remedies for a good night's sleep

Avena Sativa drops promote tranquil and uninterrupted sleep. *Arsenicum Album* 6x is good for people who have trouble sleeping between midnight and two in the morning, who have anxiety and are restless, when your brain won't stop thinking and worrying. *Arnica* 6x also calms agitated minds and can help induce sleep in people who are overly tired and can't settle down. Herbal tinctures such as Passiflora Incarnata and Melissa (take one or the other, not both) promote peace of mind and easy sleep.

If you suffer from insomnia or are not refreshed by sleep, and the above remedies don't help, you may want to consult a homeopath, herbalist, or acupuncturist. Sleeping problems often relate to emotional imbalance as well as chronic fear or anxiety about life. These practitioners consider the totality of your case, including emotional factors, and offer solutions that will not tax your body.

To promote a good night's sleep, it is best not to eat too late or to overstimulate the mind with late-night mental exertion. Think about what you do most evenings. The time before bed should be calm and peaceful, when you put aside the activities of the day. Do you give this to yourself? Or are you taxing an already overtaxed system?

If all this talk about rest and a good night's sleep strikes you as a fantasy, take a look at the demands in your life that stop you from resting or sleeping deeply. Examining your life carefully this way is a useful exercise because, in doing so, you begin to take responsibility for how you use your energy.

An active businessman I know manages on his days off to sleep till noon, getting twelve to fourteen hours of uninterrupted sleep. He says this is the only way he can keep up with the pressures of his work. When he is away from work, he doesn't waste his energy drinking, and his body rests better at night. He slows down and relaxes with his family. He eats a good meal early in the day, so he "kips out for his beauty rest" as he explains it.

MASSAGE: THREE VARIATIONS ON A THEME

Having a regular massage helps keep your body toned and your mind relaxed. We all have chronic places in our body where we store our tension: at the back of the neck, under the shoulder blades, in the jaw, at the base of the spine. A good massage therapist finds those places of chronic tension and opens them up with gentle attention and persistent effort. A good masseuse gets to know your body and is able to read it like a map, helping you let go into ease and pleasure.

Under chronic stress, muscles become hard, and even numb to feeling. Chronic tension interferes with the oxygen supply to muscles. Massage releases and soothes those chronically deprived areas, gently bringing them back to life.

Massage is an ancient therapy, dating back to early Egypt and China. In Japan, for instance, every doctor is trained in the art of massage therapy. In the West, medical and lay people have begun to recognize the powers of massage. If you have never had a massage, I highly suggest you try it. There are now many massage therapists working in beauty salons and health spas, as well as those working independently. Look for someone professionally trained or, if you have friends who get regular massages, ask for their recommendations. If you cannot afford the services of a professional on a regular basis, consider exchanging massage with a friend.

There are many forms of massage. Here, I focus on three methods I have found particularly helpful: self-massage, aromatherapy massage, and deep-tissue massage. You can decide which one works for you. Use them according to your particular need at a given time.

Self-Massage

There is a story that the warriors of Genghis Khan massaged themselves with olive oil all over their bodies, using the side of a small spoon, before going into battle to relieve tension and fear. Like those warriors, by massaging yourself you can learn where you hold your tension and help release it. Self-massage can help you relax, release tension blocks, and help you regain your vitality. A good time to do self-massage is at night before bed. Use sesame oil, olive oil, or body cream. These have healing properties and are good for your skin. Adding specific aromatic oils to this base helps balance your chakras; relaxes, stimulates, or tones your energy; and brings peace and stability to your emotions. Here are the essential oils that balance each chakra.

- *Sandalwood* for the Root Chakra

- *Jasmine* for the Sacral Chakra

- *Lemon* for the Solar Plexus

- *Rose* for the Heart Chakra

- *Blue Chamomile* for the Throat Chakra

- *Mint* for the Brow Chakra

- *Lavender* for the Crown Chakra

You can add two to three drops of oil to your bath as well as to your massage mixture. Oils can be blended; use a drop or two of each chakra oil. I make up a four-chakra oil of rose, jasmine, lemon, and chamomile for self-massage. In addition to balancing the chakra energy, it works well to open my chest if I have a cold, or soothe any tension I hold in my shoulder blades.

Begin the self-massage at your feet. Give each foot a thorough massage, going in-between the toes, stimulating the entire sole of the foot, rubbing under and around the ankle. In India, foot massage is done to help women in childbirth because Indians recognize the foot as a representation of the entire body, with every part of the body corresponding to an area on the foot. This is the premise of reflexology, a form of massage done on the foot to heal the body. The healing power of reflexology is attributed to the ability of foot massage to decongest toxins and tensions. Once you get used to working on your feet, you can use the eraser tip of a pencil or a blunted point to stimulate the points on your foot.

Next, move up the calves of the legs and knead the muscles, using your thumbs and fingers to release any knots. Give the knees a thorough massage, especially the area behind the knees. You keep the joints supple and arthritis at bay by doing this daily. If you suffer from joint problems, heat the olive oil and massage it into your joints. This is an old treatment for rheumatism and arthritis. Though it may not cure the condition, it brings soothing relief from contraction and pain.

Continue up your legs, then work your way up the front of the body, massaging your stomach in a clockwise direction. This releases deep tension in the belly which can cause constipation and block vitality in your deep organs. It is soothing and helps you relax.

Move to the right side of the body over the liver and gallbladder (right side of upper abdomen, just beneath the diaphragm) and massage this area thoroughly. This aids the flow of energy in the liver.

As a side note, if you have liver problems, you may want to use the healing liver compress devised by the famous clairvoyant Edgar Cayce. To make the compress, put castor oil (you can heat the oil slightly) on a flannel cloth, place the cloth on your abdomen in the area of your liver. Lay a piece of plastic on top of the cloth, with a heating pad or hot water bottle on top of that. Lie still for half an hour to give the healing oil time to be absorbed into the body. With a diet designed for decongestion (low in fat, with plenty of vegetables and fruit), the compresses help restore a damaged liver.

Continue the self-massage by doing your chest, heart area, and neck, then do both arms. Though it is difficult to do your back, you can rub your shoulders, hips, sacral area, buttocks, and the back of your legs. Your shoulders should be more relaxed in this position and you can rub them easily. Massage the back of your neck and your face. If you want to include your scalp, massage the oil on the top and sides of your head and leave it in overnight so that it can be absorbed. You can shampoo it out the next morning. The oil is also good for your hair.

Self-massage is self-affirming. Take an evening to give yourself a massage with a hot bath afterward. It is a way of taking care of yourself and honoring your body. Don't be strict about how often you do self-massage. Being overzealous about any routine creates more tension. Do it when you need to rest and relax. Put on some nice music, light a candle, and love yourself a little. That is a cure for tension and promotes well-being.

Aromatherapy Massage

Aromatherapy was used extensively by the ancient Egyptians over 5,000 years ago. They grew specific plants and herbs expressly for their healing oil and perfumes. When these oils are used in massage, their healing properties are delivered to your body through both smell and the skin.

Essential oils from different plants have distinct properties, and can be used to stimulate the body's energy or relax it. An aromatherapist will custom-blend oils for you, choosing those which will help heal you and also give you pleasure. If you want to mix the oils yourself, you can purchase them from health food stores and even from pharmacies. As the oils are quite concentrated, you only need a few drops of an aromatic oil in a carrier base of olive, sesame, or grapeseed oil to receive its benefits.

The following essential oils are some you might want to try:

↬ *Sandalwood* gives a luxurious sense of well-being and stability, cleanses the blood, and calms the nerves. It is associated with the Root Chakra.

✤ *Neroli* is an expensive and delicious-smelling form of orange blossom. One drop in oil or in a blend promotes pleasure and ease, and calms and stabilizes your emotions. This oil works on the Sacral Chakra.

✤ *Jasmine* is one of the most pleasurable, sensuous oils. It stimulates the Sacral Chakra to open to pleasure, ease, well-being, and sexuality.

✤ *Lemon and grapefruit* are astringent oils which help cleanse the cells. They work in a similar fashion as the citrus fruit you eat; that is, they cut through fat and stimulate the liver and gallbladder. Anyone with stomach or digestive problems can benefit from using these two oils. They also work on the Solar Plexus, where a lot of tension is stored.

✤ *Basil oil* is another rich cleanser. It works on the Solar Plexus, bringing stability and easing tension. It also cleanses and stimulates the heart.

✤ *I recommend that you buy Attar of Rose.* Though it costs more, the effects are pure bliss. This oil can cleanse the blood, tonify and relax the heart, and bring your higher senses into alignment with your energy field. It works on the Heart Chakra.

✤ *Mimosa* is an oil also used for the heart. It helps open blocked emotions. It is good for relaxation and is an antidote for stress, and is said to ease shyness and timidity.

✤ *Chamomile* is a soothing and relaxing oil that can open the Throat Chakra and help bring tranquillity to a stressed system. It has been used traditionally as a tea to soothe headaches and acid stomachs. It releases tension at the back of the neck and around the upper chest, throat, and jaw.

⤷ *Clary Sage* is a stimulant and should be used with caution. One drop in an oil base is sufficient to wake you up when you feel slow or sluggish. Sometimes I just open the bottle and take a sniff to bring clarity to my mind and emotions. It opens the Brow Chakra.

⤷ *Thyme and Rosemary* are both stimulants that work on the lungs. Along with Eucalyptus, they are excellent for decongesting the nose, throat, and weak lungs. They help restore breathing and open the spirit.

⤷ *Lavender* is the traditional oil for relaxation, often used in massage. Some aromatherapists I know put it on their pillows to ensure a good night's sleep and rub it into their temples when they have a headache. Burning a lavender-scented candle or putting a cloth with some drops of lavender oil on it near you serves as a mosquito repellent. It stimulates the Crown Chakra.

A good aromatherapy book can help you decide which oils are best for you. I do not personally ascribe to all the healing qualities that many aromatherapists attribute to essential oils. Use them for relaxation and to help you with underlying conditions that relate to stress.

I do not recommend relying on the oils to heal a serious health problem. For any serious condition, it is best to consult a medical doctor, homeopath, or acupuncturist. Treating such serious conditions with massage and aromatic oils, however, helps soothe nerves and stimulate circulation, which in itself is important in regaining health.

Deep-Tissue Massage

Deep-tissue massage refers to any method of massage in which the therapist works deeply in the muscles and tissues around the spine and joints to release energy blocks formed by chronic stress and suppressed or unresolved emotions. In body work, the body is regarded as the storehouse of the unconscious. What you don't allow yourself to experience emotionally becomes trapped in the structure of your muscles. Therefore, when blocks are released on the physical level, they also are released at a deeper emotional level.

Deep-tissue massage is used in a number of different body-work techniques. This form of massage requires time and repetition (usually a minimum of ten sessions) in order to fully release chronic blocks in the muscles and fascia (connective tissue; a fibrous membrane that attaches tissues and holds muscle together).

I have experienced excellent results from deep-tissue massage, including easing of the contraction of my feet after three sessions with my deep-tissue masseuse. She is gentle but firm and takes time to create a sense of trust between her hands and my body. If a massage therapist dives right into working on a deep level in your muscles and surrounding tissue, the muscular mass simply contracts, making clearing the blockages impossible. The body has its own natural defenses and does not open unless it feels trust.

The defensive muscular masses that limit your expression and sense of well-being were formed over many years. To suggest that they will disappear within a session or two is fantasy. It takes psychological preparation to let go of defensive patterns stored in your muscles, and a sense of attunement with the therapist who is facilitating the work.

Often during deep-tissue massage, patients experience rage, grief, anxiety, or other emotions they have suppressed over the years. They may also suddenly feel extremely tired as years of holding are released. For this reason, it is best to have a therapist who is open to dealing with these sensitive matters and can acknowledge your feelings without indulging them. This is energy that was stored in the body structure a long time ago and, though you may not know the source of the original emotion, you are familiar with the holding pattern that resulted from its suppression. It is enough to recognize what you did with your feelings and to let them go. Rather than making them significant, they need only be experienced, communicated, and released.

Choose your therapist with care, as this will be a deeply intimate, although professional, relationship you establish. If you feel that any emotional manipulation transpires between you and your therapist, find another therapist immediately. Someone who does deep-tissue massage needs a clean emotional slate and needs to honor the vulnerability of clients who put their body and souls into his or her hands. Sometimes the therapist may have all of this, but is just not a good match for you. Whenever I feel that a therapist is not tuned into me or my body, I don't return for a second massage.

Care in selection applies, of course, to any therapist you consult, but it is particularly important when you give over your body to be worked on at a deep and penetrating level. Go with what and who feels good to you and cultivate a working relationship with your therapist. They become part of your inner circle of allies.

Deep-tissue massage helps establish strong connections between your mind, body, and spirit, and reanimates your body awareness. When you release the emotions trapped in your body, you release energy that can be used for your creativity, joy, beauty, and pleasure. Many people report feeling more alive, more sexual, and more deeply in touch with themselves after deep-tissue massage.

Whenever I reach a deep emotional block in deep-tissue massage, afterward I take the homeopathic remedy *Arnica* 6x to release the shock and a hot bath to relax the muscles and restore my sense of well-being. Read the section on baths in this chapter to see if there is one that might be soothing for you after a deep-tissue massage.

OTHER BODY-WORK THERAPIES

In addition to massage, there are many other body-work techniques that can help promote relaxation, restore the energetic balance in your body, and correct structural problems or injuries that may be interfering with the clear flow of energy.

As an active, working woman who likes dancing, hiking, working out, and swimming, I need my body to support me. When I have problems with my body which limit my capacity for pleasure, I seek a reliable body therapist who can assist me in regaining full function. The therapeutic techniques in this section (cranial-sacral therapy, the Alexander Technique, and the body manipulation therapies of chiropractic and osteopathy) have served me well and play an important part in my health and beauty regime. I also have rolfing/structural integration work on a regular basis.

I once developed a frozen shoulder after a highly traumatic encounter. I felt emotionally frozen after the experience and my shoulder somatized the trauma; in other words, the unexpressed emotion took up residence in my shoulder. It became a chronic problem which was only resolved after weekly Alexander Technique sessions for many months.

This story illustrates the havoc unexpressed emotions can wreak on the body and also the need to find the therapy that works best for you. We sometimes encounter difficult situations which serve our emotional growth, but which are hard on us physically. A good body therapist can keep the body from contracting and imploding on itself. They assist us in staying open and dealing with life as it presents itself. We win every time we willingly address the needs of our body. When we give up on growth and healing, our body collapses under the weight of its own burdens and gravity takes over. We feel and look pulled down and heavy.

Use the body therapies that appeal to you. Don't get taken in by a sales pitch for a therapy that will require you to return weekly for an eternity. You may only need a few sessions. Listen to your body and trust what you experience. Your body is your friend and teacher and all therapies have a beginning and an end.

Cranial-Sacral Therapy

Cranial-sacral therapy (CST) is a gentle, noninvasive form of energy balancing which facilitates the release of deep tension in the body through palpating the deep cranial-sacral pulses of the body. It works on the principles of fluid hydraulics, in this case, the spinal fluid which bathes both the brain and spinal cord, which, in turn, feed all the nerves in the body. This fluid travels through electrical impulse stimulation moving along the nerve fibers encased in the fascia. Every part of the body is reached through these circuits, so the impact of CST is comprehensive and thorough. The cranial fluid acts as a conductor for the electrical impulses to travel throughout the body. When this fluid is balanced the sense of harmony one experiences is bliss.

These circuits respond to the lightest touch and intention of adjustment. The CST therapist applies light pressure on the bones of the cranium (skull), and along the spine, and on the feet. The touch is so gentle as to be almost imperceptible, though, in fact, the therapist is feeling this pulse of the spinal fluid and making the adjustments needed to restore its optimal flow, bringing balance and harmony to your whole system. Tension is released through the soft and gentle adjustment and balancing techniques.

The cranial-sacral therapy adjustments release areas of compression where fascia has adhered to bone and mobility is impaired. When this happens, the body has to compensate by finding new routes for energy to travel. In releasing these areas of compression, tissue is freed and mobility is restored.

Cranial-sacral therapists have generally undergone a long training that includes study in anatomy and physiology. They are taught various gentle releasing movements that ease areas of tension and bring equilibrium to the nerves and the sensorium. CST can be used by everyone and works especially well for chronic headaches and back, neck, and joint problems.

CST has been applied to newborns to correct the compression of the skull which occurs during birth. A skilled cranial-sacral therapist can gently ease the bones of the baby's cranium back into proper position. This has been found to help bring balance to the baby's cycles of respiration and sleep. Many mothers attest to their babies becoming more at ease, better tempered, and better able to adapt to a routine after just one session with a cranial-sacral therapist.

CST promotes self-correction and alignment in the body and reestablishes balance at a deep level, both of which have lasting healing effects. I personally find CST the most satisfying of body-work therapies; it induces a profound sense of peace, balance, and harmony. If you are under stress, and massage or other techniques do not produce sustained results, consider having some of this excellent work done to ease your internal tension. Some therapists combine deep-tissue massage with CST, which enhances the relaxation effect.

The Alexander Technique

In the early 1900s, a Tasmanian actor named Frederick Matthius Alexander looked for a solution to his repeatedly losing his voice onstage. After studying his posture in a three-way mirror for a long time, he realized that he was misusing movement in his head and neck. Eventually, through techniques of his own design, he was able to rectify this and never again lost his voice on stage.

Alexander came to Britain in the late 1920s and began to teach his technique, which corrects improper use of the body, thereby establishing proper posture. He taught both actors and aristocrats and started a school for children to teach them how to use their bodies correctly from an early age. His work endures and is taught throughout the United States, Britain, and Europe.

The theory behind the Alexander Technique is that improper use of the body will limit efficiency and flow of energy. A person with poor posture needs to learn how to manage his or her structure harmoniously and in relation to gravity. If a person is collapsed in the chest or diaphragm, for example, the Alexander Technique focuses on reeducating the back muscles so that they are uplifted.

The technique can lift your spirits and you feel lighter and more present in yourself when you give the body a sense of ease and freedom. The technique gives grace a physical embodiment and allows transformation to happen naturally. It frees the congestion of organs when the body has collapsed or contracted and restores the mind to its proper place of control over the body, a concept Alexander termed inhibition.

Inhibition translates as thinking about how we move and the ways in which we use our body, rather than being controlled by habit and impulse. For instance, one of my bad habits is plopping down into a chair, or giving in to gravity. The process of inhibition has directed me to sit consciously instead, lifting my head and neck up as my spine lowers toward the seat of the chair. This way my movements work to lengthen and widen my spine, and conserve vital energy which plopping into a chair dissipates downward. Inhibition makes me stop and think about how I am using my body.

Both gentle and noninvasive, the Alexander Technique is useful for correcting any dysfunction which expresses itself physically. It is excellent for people who do chronic, repetitive movements that throw the body out of alignment. Think of a violin player, for example, or a carpenter. The technique would show them how to use their body conservatively while it corrected the imbalance of their repetitive motions. If you examine how you read, work at a desk, drive your car, or rest, you will see that you have postural habits which amount to misuse and contribute to chronic fatigue and wasted energy. The Alexander Technique can help you become aware of and change these habits.

One exercise of the technique, the "lie down," is wonderfully relaxing. People with bad backs or those who feel tension in the neck and lower back after a day's work may find the "lie down" particularly beneficial. For this, you need a book two to three inches thick (about the size of a phone book) and a hard surface on which to lie down, such as the floor or a therapeutic couch. You can put on relaxing music, burn a candle, or light some incense if you choose.

Lie down with your occipital ridge at the back of your neck on the base of the book. This keeps the plane of your body even. Your knees should be up and your feet flat on the ground. Put your hands on your chest and spread your elbows out as far as they will go, so as to widen your back muscles, and then let them relax.

Lie still for twenty minutes. Let gravity work for you, instead of against you. Let everything fall back toward the ground. Let your eyes fall back in their sockets, your tongue fall back in your throat, your jaw relax, and your chest and abdomen sink into the floor. Keep letting go as you feel your muscles release. You will be recharged at the end of the twenty minutes.

This is the best exercise you can give your back when you are tired, because the spinal fluid which feeds and nourishes the discs (spongy matter) between your vertebrae is depleted when you are on your feet or sitting all day. When you are upright, the fluid is pulled down, drained by gravity. (It is also depleted by dehydration, so drinking a lot of fluid is good back therapy.) When you lie on your back, the entire spine gets bathed in spinal fluid, the discs are plumped up with the fluid, and your back muscles get a rest from holding you up and storing your tension.

I do the "lie down" often during the day when my back is tired from sitting at a desk. It helps release tension in the back and neck and can be an excellent preventative exercise for people with back trouble. If it is possible to do this at your office or at home during the day, it can save a strained back and give you strength and stamina for your day.

Body Manipulation: Chiropractic and Osteopathy

These two body manipulation therapies are excellent for transforming structure that has become dysfunctional. They work directly on the spine to realign bones creating blocks due to injury or disability.

The degrees of manipulation vary. You need to find the body manipulation technique that works best for you. I have found chiropractic effective for maintenance of the spine, but not for all conditions. For back injury, I prefer classical chiropractic adjustment, which some people object to as not gentle enough. I have weekly adjustments when I am writing a book because it keeps my spine energized and aligned. My chiropractor is an essential person in my health care plan.

Osteopaths are now using applied kinesiology to release blocks and restore energy. Applied kinesiology can be used to test for deficiencies and imbalances in the body, as well as to identify the best substance to reverse such conditions. It is useful in discovering exactly what the body requires, but the options for treatment are limited by the knowledge of the person conducting the testing. If the osteopath or other practitioner only knows about nutritional supplements, then the program they design will reflect that limitation. A practitioner who is versed in a range of therapies, including homeopathy and herbal medicine, may be more effective in treating your problems.

OTHER OPTIONS: BATHING

Bathing cleanses your body, refreshes your mind, and relaxes the spirit. Try it at the end of a hard day of work. It gives you time to muse over the events of the day and you go to bed ready to fall into slumber. Light a candle or several candles, burn your favorite incense, put on some relaxing music, and just lie back in a hot bath and unwind.

Taking a bath is my most relaxing daily ritual. I use different types of baths to ease me into pleasure and rebalance my energy. Chapter 10 covers hydrotherapy treatments offered in spas and health clubs, but the following baths are those you can do for yourself at home on a daily basis to induce serenity and relaxation.

↦ *Bicarbonate of Soda Bath:* Add two tablespoons of bicarbonate of soda to a tub of hot water. The nurse who introduced me to this bath said it takes the negative energy out of your energy field at the end of the day. She also found it the best remedy for tired feet and sore muscles. Soaking in this bath takes away tension, restores balance to your auric field, and helps you sleep well.

↦ *Sea Salt Bath:* You can buy commercial mineral bath packs or special salts from the Dead Sea which contain minerals for healing, but a plain box of sea salt purchased at the grocery store does the job. Add a quarter of a cup to a hot bath. This is good for skin problems, such as rash, eczema, or skin ulcers, that won't heal. It also cleanses the auric field and promotes peace of mind. Salt removes positive ions which clog our energy flow.

↦ *Epsom Salts Bath:* For another relaxing bath, add 1/2 cup of Epsom salts to a tub of hot water. This bath realigns your energy and helps restore your psychic energy (You can feel quite tired after taking this bath, so it is best not to do it in the daytime unless you can rest afterward.)

↦ *Arnica and Rescue Remedy Bath:* When I am really exhausted or have had a difficult day, I put one *Arnica* 6x tablet and two drops of Bach Rescue Remedy (a mixture of flower essences) into the water. This bath removes shock, bruise, and trauma from the body and helps regain emotional and physical well-being. It also is good when you are too tired and restless to sleep, and after travel.

✏ *Aromatherapy Bath:* I use Clary Sage, an aromatic oil, in my bath for energy, and Lavender for relaxation. Essential oils make a very enjoyable bath. You can add different mixtures such as geranium, lemon, basil, and jasmine oils. Each oil has its own particular property and can give you energy and stimulation, or peace, tranquillity, and refreshment. See the section on Aromatherapy Massage above for the qualities of specific oils.

SEXUALITY

The views about sexuality presented here are uniquely my own. They do not reflect any one therapy or philosophy, though they are influenced by years of bioenergetic analysis and various body therapies. I have developed these ideas through working with people for over thirty years and seeing how important sexuality is in self-discovery, energy balance, and healing.

Sexuality is your life energy concentrated in your body. Sexuality enhances your beauty and allows your body to expand, open, and delight in life. Sex is designed to give you pleasure and energetic release. Nothing relaxes you like a good orgasm. Orgasm softens the face, relaxes the muscles, and decongests the body. It stimulates your hormones and keeps your mucous membranes lubricated. Sexual release produces those precious endorphins from your brain which flood your bloodstream and contribute to you feeling good. Sexuality is such a precious gift that it should neither be taken for granted nor rejected on the grounds of age, morality, or single status. Sexuality helps you to find the beauty and wonder of your own body.

Sexuality is very personal, very pleasurable, and very necessary if we are to find who we are at a physical, emotional, and spiritual level. Taking the time to awaken your sexuality is as liberating and relaxing as any of the other things we have discussed in this chapter, probably more so. It is possibly the ultimate means of relaxation.

If you are not enjoying your sexuality, whether it is expressed singly or with a partner, you may wish to take some time to explore what makes you feel good and what delights you. Getting to know how your body responds sexually is important for your health and your emotional empowerment. Celibacy may be the way we avoid giving our vital sexual energy over to others, but that does not preclude feeling our own life force, giving it expression, and finding release for ourselves. Whether you are willing to pleasure yourself or engage your partner in sex on a regular basis is your decision. Just be aware that sexuality is a gift to be experienced, enjoyed, and valued.

Being orgasmic is not the responsibility of anyone other than yourself. You are responsible for your own orgasm and the quality of your sexual experience. I know nuns who are allowed to practice masturbation who are more in touch with their sexuality than some married women I have treated.

It is punishment not to allow pleasure to be a part of your life. Masturbation frees you from offering yourself to anyone who makes sexual advances, and it empowers you to know and love your body as a wondrous creation and instrument of pleasure. If you have trouble with the idea of masturbation, you might want to look at your attitudes about it. Do you think it is dirty? Do you think it is wrong to pleasure yourself? Where does the negativity come from? Examining your attitudes about sexuality may reveal that you believe your advancing age or physical shape or size is a reason to deny yourself participation in sexual activity, be it alone or with another.

A middle-aged friend related to me recently that her young lover told her that her "butter was richer" with age. That is a comment worth repeating. We all think it is the young who have the market on sexuality. In truth, mature women not only have the benefit of experience but, being less in need of proving their worth, can be more at ease, have more fun, and engage with greater latitude in what gives them and their partners pleasure. When the hormones have slowed down, you can really tune into your body and your energy, something that eludes you with the racing hormones of youth. Don't be deluded by advertising about the sexuality of the young. It takes time and experience to get to know your body and how it responds to pleasure. Only maturity offers us the grace and deeper expression found in orgasm as well as its spiritual essence.

Rethinking how you feel about your own sexuality can give you the permission you need to allow the sweetness of pleasure to express itself through your body. The Hindu name for the Sacral Chakra, which governs sexuality, translates as "My Own Sweet Abode." This chakra is the seat of your sexual energy and is essential to how your energy flows. To cut off your sexuality is to cut off the taproot of pleasure and life itself.

When we are tired or under stress, we find it difficult to rally to any sexual stimulation. If our minds are full of worry, plans, and racing thoughts, our body does not respond easily to its natural function of sexual expression and release. Often, we even forget that we have a body with needs for pleasure. All the techniques mentioned in this chapter will help resurrect your natural sexual energy. It is up to you to allow that energy to find expression.

Remember that dressing and looking sexy is how people seduce and entrap others. It is not saying that you are sexual, it is the promise of the delivery of your sexuality into someone else's hands. The most sexually healthy people I know are seldom overt in their outward expression of it. They don't have to be.

Find your sense of sexuality and enjoy it. Be discerning about how and with whom you share it. Don't use your sexuality as a weapon for obtaining security or power; it generally works against you and can ultimately create serious health problems. Sexuality is for your own pleasure and life enhancement. Connecting to your sexual energy is part of looking and feeling beautiful.

Chapter 6

℘ Eating for Life

Food is medicine. It feeds our cells by supplying the tissues with minerals and vitamins, and it nourishes both our hearts and minds. If we eat correctly, we let food help us heal. Food cleanses, detoxifies, fortifies, and helps with elimination. It can decongest and revivify an imperiled immune system.

On a psychological level, eating has a gratification factor that ranks above most everything but sex. In addition to pure pleasure, food gives us a sense of home and mothering. It implies good company, and festivities. Food eases emotional pain, and reminds us of a time when we were blessed with nurturers who provided for our needs and looked after us.

What we eat is an extension of how we regard ourselves and our bodies. Conscious minds eat wholesome, live foods. Eating a diet high in junk and dead foods is a sign of an unconscious mind and abuse of one's Self. People who don't feed themselves properly do not know how to be their own good mothers. Independent, responsible adults take care of themselves by managing to provide themselves with nutritious and sustaining food that strengthens both their bodies and minds.

Finding the right way to eat takes time and experimentation. The same diet does not work for everyone. Once you know what foods work best for you, you have a powerful healing tool. When you have established wholesome eating patterns, you feel much more alive and fit. Food is vital both to health and beauty. If you really care about yourself, you will learn about food and understand its healing gifts. If you want to find your beauty and maintain it, you need to nurture yourself with living food and fresh water.

I am not here to tell you what to eat to be beautiful, but only to suggest that you need wholesome, nutritious food to live and function. Without it, there is no beauty. Beauty is not a thin, half-starved anorexic face and body. This type of starvation always has an unwholesome emotional component. Our sense of ourselves is measured by what we are willing to give ourselves in terms of balance and enrichment.

FOOD FOR LIFE AND BEAUTY

It is essential that all food we put into our bodies be clean, unpolluted, and free of disease. Even this basic requirement is not easy to fulfill these days. Food is grown with the aid of dangerous pesticides which find their way into the inner membranes of fruit and vegetables; and most food we eat contains trace amounts of these chemicals. Food is also radiated to "preserve" it. This is a euphemism for mummification. Feeding an exhausted immune system with food loaded with chemicals and drugs contributes to health breakdown. Your kidneys, which are already struggling to cope with stress, have to work even harder to flush these toxins out of the body. The normal flow of energy in the liver and other organs is also compromised by these contaminants.

Processed food, which makes up a large portion of many people's diets, is full of additives. Eating food with additives is like pouring drugs down your throat. Highly processed foods strip the body of life, because they have no living substance and require effort to digest. Canned food has all of its life force drained out of it and is thought to be a contributor to Alzheimer's because of traces of aluminum found in the brain of those suffering from this devastating condition.

You can see the importance of choosing your food carefully. The more life force your food has, the more healing energy available for your body. You cannot get vitality from dead, highly processed, and chemically treated food. Eating organically grown food supports your body in maintaining the high energy levels you want and need. A good diet feeds your beauty and health.

I recently treated a young woman with severe acne who was lovely in all other respects. She is a rising star in her company, a friendly, open person, with a wonderful outlook on life and a love of sports.

I suggested a homeopathic remedy but especially asked her to focus on changing her diet. She ate mostly canned foods, take-out pizza, and a lot of chocolate and bread. She did not have sound mothering instincts and needed to learn how to look after herself.

I instructed her to eat only live food, avoid dairy and wheat for three months, and eat all the fresh fruit and vegetables she could manage. Within three months, her body was detoxified and her stagnant liver, often the source of acne problems, was flushing properly. Her complexion, which had been a problem for years, cleared up completely.

What emerged was a confident beauty who went out and bought some stunning clothes, had fun with her friends, and eventually met a man who became her lover and partner. I saw the transformation take place and delighted in it. In effect, she began to grow up and take responsibility for herself and nurture herself properly.

It takes commitment to improve your diet. I equate the commitment to eating well to having a sound philosophy in life. Your life philosophy gives you a foundation for looking after yourself; it helps you hold your experiences in a context you can understand and keeps chaos at bay. Eating well provides you with a physical foundation for looking after yourself; your body receives food in a consistent manner and in a healthy form which takes the strain off your digestive system and optimizes nutritive value and assimilation. Just as your life philosophy can be a source of comfort and support in difficult times, good food is something you can count on as a medicine to help keep your spirits up and your body functional.

FEEDING YOUR CHAKRAS AND ORGANS

Specific foods have an affinity to each of your chakras, or energy centers. Eating those foods strengthens the energy flow of that chakra. As the chakras feed energy to our organs, these foods will also strengthen the corresponding organ. For example, the kidneys are the organs associated with the Sacral Chakra. Orange foods such as carrots and pumpkin feed this energy center, so eating carrots and pumpkin will strengthen both your kidneys as well as your Sacral Chakra energy. If you know one chakra needs specific attention, feed it what it will thrive on for a week and see if you notice any difference in your energy.

Juicing is an invaluable part of a health and beauty regime, and is a quick way to deliver chakra-supporting foods. You can make chakra drinks from many of the foods discussed in the sections to follow. Try to avoid combining fruits and vegetables in one juice mixture. The body breaks them down differently, so it is best to ingest them separately. Eat fruits in the morning and vegetables in the afternoon or early evening.

Make sure the fruits and vegetables you use are fresh, unradiated, and free of contaminants. Old or radiated fruits and vegetables have no life force. Fresh, pure juices have healing power. They give you, in a highly concentrated form, the radiant energy of the food from which they are made. Juices are rich in vitamins and minerals and feed your body in a way that no prepared food can. They can give you an almost immediate lift when you are tired. In addition to providing energy and vitality, juices aid in detoxifying the body, cleansing the bowels, and decongesting organs. As you detoxify the body, your complexion will clear up and your aches and pains will start to disappear.

The following are suggested combinations of juices for your health and pleasure:

- Strawberry, orange, mango, papaya, and lemon

- Watermelon, grape, and kiwi

- Orange, pineapple, and lemon

- Grapefruit, orange, and pineapple

- Lemon, peach, passion fruit, and mango

- Orange, grapefruit, and blueberry

- Tomato, carrot, and cabbage

- Carrot, celery, and fennel

- Tomato, lemon, and carrot

- Spinach, cabbage, and tomato

- Fennel, cabbage, and celery

Experiment to find which combinations please your taste buds. Juice can serve as one meal in the day. If you are fasting, you can juice all your meals and have a wonderful detoxification and healing regime for a few days. Juice fasting for longer periods is not advisable, unless you are very ill and need a total detoxification, which should only be done under the care of a qualified health practitioner.

The Root Chakra: Earthy and Red Foods Full of Minerals

Food for the Root Chakra center comes from inside the earth. Thus, root vegetables, such as beets, feed this vital center of life energy and help you ground yourself. Other Root Chakra foods are legumes (peas and beans), grains, and cereals. Root Chakra foods are the dietary staples in most countries where the highly refined and dead food of industrialized society has not taken over.

You can use beets in soups, juice, and salads; grate them raw and combine them with oil and lemon for a salad, cook them as a soup with added yogurt, a hard-boiled egg, or boiled potato, or juice them with carrot and celery for a three-chakra drink (red, orange, and yellow are the colors of the first three chakras). Whole-grain brown rice is a highly nourishing Root Chakra food. It is said to be the most balanced food substance you can eat, consisting as it does of two parts yang (masculine principle) to three parts yin (feminine principle). Cooking up large pots of rice, following the ancient tradition of two parts water to one part rice, gives you a base for adding vegetables, fish, chicken, or meat, if you wish.

Brown rice can stop food cravings, stabilize the bowels, and purify the blood. Some people fast on it for ten days to purify their systems. Again, the result of detoxifying is a soft and beautiful complexion, as impurities are eliminated from the body. This fast should be done only when you need to purify your system. It should not become another fad diet. If you have serious medical problems, consult a holistic nutritionist before attempting such a fast.

Other grains that give life-sustaining energy are bulgur wheat, millet, corn, oats, and couscous. Eating oats each morning, either raw or as porridge, provides hours worth of stable nutrition and energy. Oats with sweetened soy milk, raisins, grated apple, and honey is the most satisfying breakfast I know. It is not fattening and provides excellent roughage and nutrition. If you buy organic oats, you avoid additives. Many packaged breakfast cereals contain high amounts of both sugar and sodium, so check the label of any cereal you buy. Grains provide excellent nutrition, and serve as a base for whatever else you choose to add to your diet. Making them a staple in your diet eliminates the desire to binge, starve, or be fickle about food. It creates a strong, stable way of eating which can be maintained easily, inexpensively, and with excellent benefit to your health.

All legumes (also called pulses) are solidly grounding for the spirit. In the Middle East, lentil soup and cooked beans puréed with onions, garlic, and olive oil are staples for workers, giving them great energy for the day. These foods are mentioned in the Bible and are traditionally known to provide excellent nourishment, as they contain both carbohydrates and protein.

Other root vegetables besides beets are carrots, onions, and garlic. Garlic and onions are medicines in themselves, purifying the blood and stimulating sexuality. Rutabagas, parsnips, and turnips are also good root vegetables. They can be added to a vegetable stew or cooked lightly on their own.

Red foods also provide Root Chakra energy. Tomatoes, strawberries, red currants, and raspberries contain trace elements of iron, which feeds your root energy. Watermelon is so cleansing that you can fast on it in summer for a quick clean-out. It purifies the blood and has a high sugar content which will keep you going during a fast. Watermelon, strawberries, and raspberries can be added to a Root Chakra juice drink.

Red meat, if it is from organically raised cows, is excellent for nourishing the life force. If you are very weak, ill, or run-down and in danger of becoming ill, meat can revitalize you. Too much meat creates toxicity, but in small amounts it nourishes your blood and gives you energy which is hard to obtain from any other food. If you eat meat, use only meat uncontaminated by drugs. Fresh meat is preferable, as freezing depletes life force.

Dairy products are Root Chakra foods as well. There are conflicting opinions about whether eating dairy is healthy. Excessive intake of dairy promotes mucus production in the throat, lungs, and intestines. In the latter, the mucus coats the intestinal lining and can interfere with its detoxifying functions and its ability to protect the body against microbes. Some people have difficulty digesting dairy products and others are allergic to them.

For those who have no problem with dairy products, they are a reliable source of protein and can be a staple for vegetarians. Managing a balance with dairy is important, however. You don't want to clog up your system, especially if you have spent time detoxifying.

The best dairy products are those that contain large amounts of lactobacillus (beneficial intestinal bacteria) such as live cultured yogurt, kefir, buttermilk, and hard white cheese. People with lactose intolerance are better off using nondairy products such as soy and tofu, which are high in protein.

It is a good idea to be tested for dairy and wheat intolerance, as so many people suffer from these allergies. Wheat, which has been a staple of the human diet for thousands of years, is now genetically engineered so that the body has difficulty processing it without reactions. I have seen many migraines, skin allergies, and cases of chronic constipation clear up simply by removing wheat and dairy from the diet.

The Sacral Chakra: Water Awareness and Orange Foods

The Sacral Chakra regulates the fluids in the body. Since our bodies comprise over 80 percent water, this chakra's function is vital to body stabilization. Understanding the importance of water and what it can do to stimulate and balance this chakra will assist you in your health and beauty care. Let's start by looking at the nature of the kidneys, which are the organs associated with this chakra.

The kidneys function in many ways to preserve our life force. They are thought to be the seat of our immunity. They can become tense and blocked with fear and aggression, when our life is threatened, or when we are shocked. One of their primary functions is to manufacture urine and filter impurities and toxins from the lymph and other plasma type fluids. They can, like the rest of the body, become dehydrated from lack of water.

The adrenal glands, situated atop the kidneys, produce adrenaline. This hormone is vital to activity, self-preservation, and our engagement with life. The release of adrenaline, known as fight or flight response, is triggered by any perceived threat, real or imagined. The flooding of adrenaline into the bloodstream is designed to give us super-charged energy to combat the threat. Adrenaline pumps whenever we get excited, flowing into our blood and stimulating our nerves and senses. It raises our blood pressure and "wires us up." It is the boost we get during drama and crisis.

A fast-paced, high-stress lifestyle keeps us in this fight or flight response almost continually. Some people become addicted to the adrenaline rush. Those who constantly need to be charged are unconsciously seeking the thrill of adrenaline coursing in their blood. Too many or continual fight or flight responses weakens the vitality of the kidneys and leave us weakened and drained. Constant stress, drama, and crisis burn through our supply of adrenaline. The adrenal glands cannot keep up with the demand and become exhausted and weaken the kidneys as well. When our jobs or schedules push us to the brink, our relationships break down, or we have dire financial problems, our fears, tensions, and constant striving drain the kidneys and adrenal glands. Rest and recuperation is needed to restore them.

Keeping the kidneys tonified and strong should be a conscious act. The way we do this is to nourish them by drinking pure water, free of contaminants. High levels of sodium in water weaken the kidneys as well as the heart. Fluoride in water can damage the inner walls of the veins and blood vessels, cause herniation and varicose veins, and negatively affect mental and emotional states. Spring water from deep artesian wells is best.

Drinking pure water lubricates the joints, feeds the blood, and helps the kidneys discharge impurities from the system. It helps combat fatigue and keeps the skin hydrated, which is a natural preventative of wrinkling and aging. Water is life, and drinking it supplies the medium most suited to feeding our cells.

There is a doctor in India who claims he can cure many diseases using drinking water alone. He cites dehydration as a source of back problems, which arise when the spinal fluid cannot sufficiently feed the tissue around the vertebral discs. According to this doctor, two to three liters of water a day will nourish the body and stop deterioration. Beauty therapists maintain that drinking enough water can retard the aging process.

Make sure you drink between 8 to 10 glasses of water at room temperature on a daily basis.

If you find it difficult to drink water in the winter or in cold climates, drink it in the form of herbal tea. Nettle tea is cleansing, as is mint and even plain boiled water. Caffeine drinks, such as coffee and black tea, do not count as your water intake. They are diuretics, which means they are dehydrating, so you actually have to drink even more water if you drink coffee or tea. In addition, caffeine produces a flush of adrenaline which then leaves the body depleted of energy and sends the coffee drinker in search of more caffeine to raise his energy level.

Whenever you are under stress, drink water. It irrigates the body and flushes accumulating toxins out of your kidneys, preventing the congestion that can occur during the overload of stress. The area under your eyes reveals how well or poorly your kidneys are functioning. If you have dark circles or puffiness, it means that your kidneys are congested. This could be from repeated stress, lack of sleep, or food that is too rich and difficult to digest.

Treat your kidneys with love and care. They are the seat of your ancestral family energy. In Chinese medicine, this is called ancestral *Chi* and it is the foundation of your life force. The energy you inherit from your ancestors may be strong and solid energy which you can tap into when you are under pressure. Known as the Seas of Reserve, this energy is especially stored for any life-threatening situations so that you can draw on it.

If you have constant crises in your life, you are drawing on this vital supply of energy which you should protect and keep for a time when you really need it. If you use crisis as a way of rousing yourself and getting a response from others, you may want to reconsider the value of peace in your life. All dramas and crises wear you down because they burn this very precious ancestral fuel. Preserving your life force with healthy routines, good food, and plenty of water will help you experience your natural beauty as well as keep your reserve tanks of energy full for years to come.

Orange Food for the Sacral Chakra

Orange foods stimulate the Sacral Chakra. These foods are rich in minerals and vitamins and fortify this center of life energy which controls movement, pleasure, well-being, and abundance.

Oranges, the most obvious orange food, provide natural vitamin C which we need to strengthen our immunity and keep our blood pure; vitamin C acts as an astringent, helping to break down lipids and fats in the blood. Oranges are wonderful as juice and to eat raw. They should be eaten raw and soon after being cut, in order to maintain their vitamin content, which is depleted a mere half-hour after the orange is cut open. So don't make a large jug of juice to keep in the refrigerator, but squeeze the oranges right before drinking.

Orange juice provides quick energy, but too much orange juice can make the complexion blotchy and some people's digestive system are so delicate and allergenic that they can't tolerate this fruit because of its high acid content. It can cause irritation to the gut lining and should, as with all foods, be used in moderation.

Other orange fruits are papaya (which contains papain, a digestive enzyme), mango, passion fruit, apricot, melons, and tangerines. Any mixture of these orange fruits can stimulate the cleansing of the intestinal wall and aid in good elimination. They are excellent foods for the Sacral Chakra.

All vegetables from the pumpkin and squash family are good nourishment for Sacral Chakra energy. When you are under stress, they can give you needed fortification, as they coat the myelin sheath (insulation) of nerves and thus serve to pacify the nervous system. Pumpkin is rich in germanium and other trace minerals, inexpensive, and, if you are a gardener, easy to grow. It can be used as a base for stews, soups, and pies. A tasty stew can be made with garbanzo beans, onions, garlic, and stewed pumpkin; add parsley, celery, and spices for added flavor.

Carrots, if they are organic, are a powerful healing food, because they contain enormous quantities of vitamin A. Carrots can be juiced, grated in salads, or cooked lightly. Their life force is best kept when they are eaten raw. Carrots can be juiced with beets, orange, apple, celery, and any other vegetables with one fruit, such as apple, for sweetener, to create a delicious drink that is full of energy. Excessive amounts of carrot juice can cause vitamin A toxicity, however, so don't overdo a good thing. Carrot juice is a central component in the Gerson diet (developed by Max Gerson) for treating cancer. It has a special property which is effective in discouraging chaotic growth of cancer cells.

Another excellent Sacral Chakra fruit is apricot. Containing vitamins and minerals that stimulate rejuvenation and health, apricots have rich healing properties. Laetrile, a substance used to fight cancerous growths, is derived from apricot kernels. The oil from the kernels smoothes and softens the skin; it is used in many beauty products. According to the Law of Signatures, which helps you identify the healing properties of a plant by looking at its shape and color, you can see what its healing properties are. When you see the soft, lustrous color and texture of the apricot, you can imagine what it will do for your complexion.

Fish makes sense as a food for the Sacral Chakra, because this center controls water balance in the body. The Hindu symbol for this chakra is a type of crocodile that protects this vital energy center. Salmon and pink trout particularly nourish the Sacral Chakra. The ancient Celts considered salmon the fish of sacred wisdom. Salmon is now used as a homeopathic remedy to aid in fertility, which is governed by this center. Salmon gives a tremendous boost to the life force. Think of the salmon spawning up river and you have an idea of the intelligence, life-preserving instincts, and vitality of this fish. Unfortunately, salmon have been so overfished in the wild that most of the fish you buy comes from salmon farms, a method contrary to the free, roaming nature of the fish.

Fowl is also Sacral Chakra food. Buy only free-range poultry, because it will be chemical free as well as more tasty. A free-range chicken or turkey provides a high level of nutrition. Turkey is one of the highest sources of protein of all animal foods.

Vitamins, Supplements, and Herbs
Related to the Sacral Chakra

Vitamins and other supplements come under the Sacral Chakra food supply, because they work directly on physical vitality. Supplements have become a major business. We are told that because food is so contaminated and vitamin deficient, we need supplements to keep us healthy. This is a half truth.

There are two things wrong with glutting our bodies with vitamins and other supplements: we take away the body's natural ability to absorb. Whenever we have to " kick start" our systems with vitamins or medication we stop our body's natural ability to function. The body may not be able to absorb the highly enriched and concentrated substances. If our systems are too weak and congested to assimilate the nutrients, no amount of enriched supplements poured into us will make a difference to our nutrition. All those unabsorbed vitamins and minerals are just flushed out of the body via the urine. You can spend a fortune on supplements without achieving results. It is more important to address the body's weakened ability to break down and absorb food. Please read the section on Energetic Medicine for more information.

It is better to build the body's natural immunity by creating balance in the system. This is done best with homeopathy and acupuncture and, occasionally, with herbs. (For more information on these natural healing methods, see Chapter 8.) Begin the process of healing by eating wholesome food as your best source of vitamins, rather than immediately popping supplements. Beauty is based on balance.

There are times, however, when supplements are useful: during periods of change and stress, to regain lost strength after an illness, or to fortify an immune system in danger of breaking down. When you are under stress, for example, you need additional vitamins B and C, which help strengthen the nerves and keep the tissues irrigated. There are many books on vitamins and minerals which can help you determine what you need and how you can treat deficiency.

Supplements should be used as a booster to the body's natural healing process, never taken continuously over a long time. Excessive or prolonged dosages can harm the body. I advise my patients to take supplements for only three months in winter, when their bodies work extra hard to stay strong. I ask them to avoid using synthetic vitamins. The body is better able to absorb natural, organic supplements.

Unfortunately, many people use supplements as a substitute for lifestyle changes they should implement for their health. Slowing down, eating live foods, getting enough exercise are all factors in health management. From a mental point of view, when you take a lot of supplements, you are making the statement that you feel weak, vulnerable, and unable to handle the pressures of your life. Wouldn't it be better to address the problem directly than to project healing power into a vitamin or other supplement?

Homeopaths are encountering more patients who are toxic from overdosing on vitamins. They are stripping away the mucous lining of their digestive tracts with enormous amounts of vitamin C. We have actually started to antidote this poisoning in homeopathy by giving potentized vitamin C, in keeping with homeopathy's principle of treating "like cures like." This remedy restores the mucous membranes and helps the patient regain his or her own internal cleansing faculties.

Herbs also feed the Sacral Chakra. They are strongly alkaline in nature and you need a certain level of vitality to digest them. I prefer herbs to vitamin supplements because they are closer to the natural state and can be accepted into the body more readily. Herbs can work well to cleanse the body and restore vitality.

All supplements and herbs work in substantial, material form. This means they are not diluted, or potentized, as are homeopathic remedies derived from the same plant, which means herbs are not as powerful as homeopathics. The effects of a homeopathic remedy can last for several weeks, even months, and its healing properties work to establish balance without the strong effects of highly alkaloid substances. You may want to consider homeopathy rather than supplements or herbs.

Some people are now taking herbal weight loss supplements to metabolize food faster and speed up weight loss. It has been found that many of these supplements contain the substance ephedra, or ma huang, the Chinese herb. It suppresses the appetite while stimulating metabolism. This substance has been the cause of death and over one thousand adverse reactions have been documented. Side effects, according to *Prevention's Guide to Healing Herbs*, are increased blood pressure, nervousness, heart palpitations, headaches, dizziness, and vomiting. Reader be warned. This is not the way to lose weight effectively.

The Solar Plexus: Food to Feed Your Power Center
People who suffer from low confidence and lack of empowerment often develop health problems in the stomach, gallbladder, liver, and pancreas, the organs fed by the power chakra, or Solar Plexus. On a physical level, this energy center governs food digestion and absorption. On a psychic plane, its energy works on the digestion and assimilation of ideas.

Dysfunction is the inability to digest certain foods, as well as the symptoms of heartburn, gas, or stomach pain. If a person doesn't feel he or she is loved in the right way and is too timid to address this issue, he or she generally develops problems in the gallbladder. Stones form, which can be painful and impede and congest that organ.

Drug use, long-term bad eating habits, and suppressed anger can all congest the liver and create a stasis which blocks the flow of bile. When you take synthetic vitamins, alcohol, drugs, or HRT (hormone replacement therapy) or any other hormones, the liver, which is the body's toxin filter, has to process them. When you burden the liver with these substances, you take away its normal job of detoxifying the blood.

The liver is responsible for breaking down estrogen in the body. As women age and their menstrual cycle comes to an end, estrogen is no longer produced in the ovaries; what remains of this hormone in the body is produced in the adrenal glands. The breakdown of this hormone happens in the liver and this organ must be strong enough to do its job. A weak liver cannot eliminate estrogen efficiently. Excessive estrogen in the blood contributes to a series of problems and may be a causative factor in breast cancer.

Fatty, sugary, and chemical-laden foods block the liver and gallbladder from functioning properly. Alcohol is such a refined sugar that it can destroy the liver when used excessively over long periods of time.

Foods which feed the Solar Plexus energy center are those which cleanse and fortify the liver and gallbladder. Foods rich in vitamins A and C and minerals act as liver tonics. All vegetables are good for the liver, as are butter (in small quantities) and olive oil. Greens cleanse the liver by helping to break down fatty deposits. Lemons and grapefruit are also natural cleansers, reducing the level of lipids in your blood. Grapefruit is an excellent food for losing weight because it helps break down fatty deposits in the liver and gut lining.

Feeding the liver sufficient quantities of protein helps to keep it strong. Eggs are a Solar Plexus food, providing they come from free-range chickens or ducks. High in cholesterol, they should be eaten only occasionally. When you have been ill, they provide a natural strength which the body absorbs easily.

Sunshine is food for the Solar Plexus. The Sun is the central planet of this chakra, and sunshine actually stimulates the digestion of food. It is important to have regular, but moderate exposure to sunshine. It creates vitamin D and strengthens the system. Evidence of this lies in the fact that summers in which there is little or no sun produce flu epidemics the following winter.

In addition to supporting your liver by what you eat, there are liver flushes used by herbalists to nourish the function of this vital organ. I recommend Dr. Christopher's liver flush recipes (found in most herbal books). A simple and effective liver flush consists of the juice of half a lemon and a teaspoon of honey mixed in warm water and taken first thing in the morning. This revitalizes and tonifies a torpid liver.

If the liver is not functioning optimally, a vertical line appears between the eyebrows. This is the liver line and can indicate a poor diet, drug or alcohol abuse, or HRT. A turbulent emotional life can be read from this line as well. People who have a liver line are easily irritated and angry, but store their anger inside. Physically, they often have a problem with chronic constipation.

All this from one line on the face! If you continue to abuse the liver, the line can become a groove which is extremely unattractive and unresponsive to beauty treatments. You can plaster it with makeup, even have collagen injections, but stress on your liver will make the line deeper and more apparent.

Green Foods for the Heart Chakra

As we age, our hearts bear the strain of all our difficult challenges and emotionally painful experiences. Emotions, changes, and loss weaken the heart as much as rich food and smoking can. Today, people are obsessed with their cholesterol levels and blood pressure. The underlying fear is that if they don't look after themselves, they will die. This anxiety and the negative thoughts that go along with it, also put a strain on the heart. The heart enjoys ease, pleasure, laughter, and smiles. It loves lightness and frivolity. It longs for expression of its deepest qualities, which are love and joy.

The heart and blood require pure and natural foods, however. By giving our heart the food it needs, we can support it in thriving under the strains and pains of life. The heart does well with a low-sodium, low-sugar, and low-fat diet. The blood does well with food rich in iron and potassium, such as legumes (pulses), beans, and vegetables. Meat can promote strength and resiliency in people with weak hearts, but only if it is fresh and free of chemical preservatives.

Green foods and algae are excellent for the heart and blood. They help keep the body calm and supply ready energy. Green foods act as a natural diuretic, promoting drainage so a weakened heart does not become congested with damaging, saline-rich fluids. Watercress, abundant in ferrum sulfate, provides triple the recommended daily iron intake. Celery, parsley, cilantro, and cumin are rich in potassium. A broth made with zucchini, parsley, celery, and spinach and blended with yogurt can be served hot or cold and fortifies the system by giving you enough potassium to take you through a stressful day. It maintains the electrolyte balance of the pericardium (membrane around the heart) and can aid in cleansing the venous blood as it returns to the heart to be oxygenated.

The lungs are also governed by the Heart Chakra. If the lungs are weak, avoid dairy products. They congest the lungs and are hard for the body to break down. Use them sparingly and only when the weather is warm so that they are more easily digested. Soy milk can provide protein and calcium without the mucus-producing side effect of cow's milk. Calcium feeds the heart and keeps the nerves soothed. Ginger is a good food for heating the lungs, especially in cold weather. Hot fluids, soups, warm drinks, and hot water are also good for the lungs.

If you have a desire for a certain food, trust that there is something your body needs that this food contains. When we are trying to create healthy eating, we want to give our hearts and blood the most nutritious food possible. But sometimes, soul food or the food we had in childhood gives the heart a moment of happiness that may be more enriching than a dietetically correct meal.

For heart health, avoid caffeine tea, coffee, and sugar. These tax the heart and can contribute to palpitations and angina. Sugar weakens the circulatory system and venous walls and causes problems to an already damaged heart. Cigarette smoking may be the single worst thing anyone with heart or lung disease can do to themselves. The deleterious effects of smoking should be apparent to anyone seeking health and beauty.

Food for the Throat Chakra

There are a few foods that feed the Throat Chakra. Honey is one, and can be used as a sugar substitute to satisfy your sweet tooth.

Dates and other dried fruits are also sweet alternatives to sugar. Unlike sugar, they do not cause mucus buildup, which can block the throat and sinuses.

If you suffer from sore throats, a mixture of fresh lemon juice and a spoonful of honey soothes the lining of the throat and helps it to heal. If you have to sing or speak publicly, avoid dairy products and chocolate. These will produce mucus immediately and can clog your throat.

The Throat Chakra controls substance abuse, so foods for this center need to reflect balance in nutrition and quantity. People who abuse their bodies with drugs or alcohol often pour junk food and chemicals (processed food with additives, preservatives, and agricultural pesticide residues) into their systems as well. If they aren't concerned about damage from substances, they are unlikely to consider diet. Weakened Throat Chakras are made weaker by drugs, cigarettes, junk food, and alcohol. This is the center of the will. When we pour junk into our systems, we don't give the will an opportunity to grow.

Food for the Brain: Feeding the Third Eye

The best brain foods are considered to be almonds, walnuts, fish, and eggs. They bring nutrition to the whole person, but are also rich in the trace minerals (such as germanium and molybdenum) and other substances which act as catalysts to the functioning of the brain. Over two thousand years ago, Aristotle spoke of the power of tea and almonds to supply the brain with food. Six almonds are said to be the daily food of thinkers. Tea cleanses the blood and helps keep the mind alert. Fish has traditionally been regarded as the food for wisdom and intelligence. We also feed the brain when we give it the fluid supply it needs, and the balance of oils, trace minerals, and glucose (sugar) that keeps it fueled.

In my clinical homeopathic practice when I see difficult children with behavioral or learning problems, I know that they are improperly fed, especially in the mornings. With insufficient breakfast, their minds won't be active and alert at school. Learning takes energy and it has to come from a physical source. Eating cold Pop-Tarts on the school bus doesn't supply that energy.

As adults, many of us, especially weight-conscious women, have a breakfast of coffee. Others start their day with a pastry. If our minds don't have the fuel to work, how are we going to get through the day fulfilling our tasks and making decisions that may affect ours and other people's lives? Too many people fail to realize the importance of supplying the brain with fuel so that it can function properly. Refined sugar depletes brain energy and can cause hypoglycemia (low blood sugar) and spaciness. Spaced-out, hypoglycemic (high blood sugar) people make bad decisions. They are starved of energy. Instead of eating sugar and coffee, get a good start on the day by fueling the brain with a wholesome breakfast of oats, other grain cereal, or whole-grain bread and butter.

Herbal extracts of guarana, gingko biloba, and ginseng are known to keep the brain focused by raising the blood pressure and increasing the supply of oxygen to the brain. They should be used sparingly, only when you have an excess of work or must stay awake and alert to complete the job. Otherwise, prolonged use diminishes function.

Feeding the Crown Chakra: Fasting to Open the Spirit

Providing food for the spirit does not involve physical feeding. Rather, the energy of the Crown Chakra is strengthened by fasting. Traditionally, fasting has been done by mystics and other spiritual seekers to nourish their spirituality and open their hearts and minds to the luminous mysteries of the universe.

Fasting can be used to purify the body as well as the soul, but should be undertaken carefully, preferably with a nutritionist's or healer's guidance, at least the first time you do it. Prolonged and repeated fasting is harmful to the body. To fast on only water is also hard on your system and can leave you energetically depleted.

Careful fasting is done with a combination of fruit and vegetable juices, water, and teas prepared from herbs. Vegetable broth is also used. There are a wide variety of fasts and, if fasting interests you, you need to find what works best for you.

I try to fast four times a year, on or near the fall and spring equinoxes and the summer and winter solstices. At these times, the earth energy is shifting and the spirit is in tune with the deeper meaning of these cyclical changes. For all but one fast, I fast for no more than four or five days. I always try to give myself the time for solitude, prayer, and reflection. These are sacred times, an opportunity to reflect on my path, on what happened to me in the season passing, and on what I wish to accomplish in the coming season.

During the winter, I like to do a brown rice fast for ten days, the longest fast I do. It purifies my system after the Christmas glut and helps to increase my sensitivity and awareness. The fast prepares me to face the cold months ahead with vitality and a fortified immune system.

In the spring, I fast on water, juice, and vegetable broth for four days to cleanse my system and prepare my energy for the new life of spring. I feel good doing this fast just as the new shoots of spring are emerging from the ground. I try to get plenty of fresh air and exercise at this time as well. All of this helps me feel renewed and ready for life.

At the fall equinox when I have the good fortune to be in a sunny climate and the grapes are ripe, I like to fast on grapes and water. I eat a maximum of one pound of grapes a day, and preferably ones that haven't been chemically sprayed. This is a wonderful cleansing fast and I am always full of energy from the sugar of the grapes. This fast has been known to help eliminate cancerous growths and purify diseased systems for many people. There are several books written about the grape cure which are worthwhile reading.

I also like to fast on the juice of beets, carrots, apples, and celery for three days, along with a lot of hot herbal tea and warm water. This fast gives my system a rest from all the activity of the summer and sets me up for the approaching cold weather.

Fasting heightens your awareness. Smells become acute, your hearing opens up, and your body has a chance to discharge toxins that have accumulated with stress. It is not advisable to fast when you are under pressure and need to be active and engaged with people or projects. Along with toxins, fasting can release deep emotional stress that has accumulated, bringing these emotions to the surface. I often have a good weep when I fast.

Fasting brings my spirit closer to my conscious mind. I like to be alone for the times I fast, and require long periods of silence and tranquillity. It is a time of inner resolution, rejuvenation, and peace. I sleep long and deeply and emerge from the fast with my sense of purpose renewed.

There are books on fasting by holistic nutritionists who can guide you through a fast. When the body has been cleansed, often skin ailments, arthritis, and other congestive health problems vanish or are much better. Fasting is used, under controlled supervision, for the treatment of cancer, as the Gerson method has proved successfully. Fasting is contraindicated for heart problems, however.

FOOD, HERBS, AND SUPPLEMENTS FOR
AGING AND MENOPAUSE

As there are foods that support each chakra and organ, there are foods that nurture the body and help retard the aging process and the imbalance which comes with menopause.

Think of food as medicine and you will approach eating with more awareness and consideration for your body's needs. Whenever the body experiences intense periods of stress or life change, it needs foods that are rich in potassium, protein, and calcium. Finding the right combination of foods which support change and provide maximum healing for the overworked body takes time and thought. It is part of learning to manage any change that comes with life.

In regard to overeating and undereating, remember we are looking for balance, because that is where our beauty can thrive. Repeated dieting destroys beauty. A face wizened from starvation shows the ravages of age more quickly. Fissures form in the cheeks, the liver line enlarges, and small wrinkles form around the mouth and eyes, indicating estrogen deficiency and liver dysfunction.

As the body ages, it does thicken and adds girth. Cells become thin and flat and lose their moisture and elasticity. It is important at any age to eat a healthy, wholesome diet that supports you in your life and work, but it becomes even more important as you get older. While a young woman can get away with living on candy bars, coffee, and cigarettes, maturity demands that you feed the vitality of your body with natural energy. The days of bingeing, starving, and malnutrition are over if you want to maintain high levels of beauty and grace. Your appearance benefits from healthy eating and it can make the difference between feeling well or suffering from such problems as bloating, gas, sweats, allergies, and depression.

As I have emphasized throughout this chapter, organically raised, natural foods are the best. If the work you do means you often have to eat in restaurants and hotels, choose the foods that are easy to digest and are water-soluble, such as fruit and vegetables. Be sure to drink as much as eight glasses of mineral water (not in aluminum cans) daily to filter out the toxins that are bound to be in restaurant foods. Drinking plenty of water is important at all times, not just when you are eating a less than optimal diet. Water stops the cells from dehydrating and helps keep the bowels regular, which means emptying several times daily.

A healthy diet is part of what all beautiful women cultivate. Understanding the healing properties of foods gives you the advantage of being able to draw on certain foods when you need them. It is good to know what foods calm, which ones strengthen, which ones stimulate. Take responsibility for what you put into your body and you may be surprised at how well your body responds to your care and kindness.

For women going through menopause, it is important to eat protein. If you are carnivorous, eat one meal of protein daily. This keeps the liver active and allows it to break down estrogen in your body. If you are vegetarian, you need to increase the amount of tofu and other soy products in your diet at this time of your life.

Foods rich in B vitamins, such as soy, oats, whole-grain brown rice, and eggs keep your nerves strong.

Calcium deficiency is often a worry for menopausal women because the bones lose their density and porosity at this time of life. Weight-bearing exercise strengthens the bones, and supplements and increased levels of soy products can fulfill your calcium needs. Three cups of soy milk daily provide extra stamina and meet the daily calcium requirement. You can use soy milk by itself, on your cereal, in tea, or blended with honey or fruit. Hot flashes are another concern of menopausal women. Ginseng and vitamin B6 taken daily for three to four months stopped my hot flashes within a few months of taking them. Having since learned homeopathy, I now take homeopathic estrogen and progesterone. These can be obtained from a homeopathic pharmacy; the recommended potency is 6x taken three times daily. Women are always thankful for this bit of information, which helps transform menopause into a creative and active time rather than a time of suffering and hardship.

The following supplements and herbs also help promote stability and well-being during menopause:

⇝ *Evening primrose oil, borage oil, wild yam, dong quai (angelica):* work on hormonal balance, providing essential fatty acids and enzymes which stimulate hormonal production.

⇝ *Agnus-castus (vitex), hypericum, magnesium:* work on the nerves, providing emotional and mental stability.

⇝ *Licorice root, dandelion root, milk thistle:* cleanse the liver and keep the liver's portal system of venous flow efficient.

Many of the above herbs are found in homeopathic form as

well. Homeopathic remedy dosages are minimal, as compared to the everyday dosing required by their herbal counterparts.

Like beauty products, various other supplements come and go as the anti-aging flavor of the month. I am completely satisfied with the results of using homeopathy, acupuncture, and the supplements I mention above to ease menopause and maintain life vitality. Be cautious of any product promising to reduce effects of aging. Regaining your health and vitality takes time and consistency. There are no miracle cures. If you need nutritional consultations seek a mature, healthy, and beautiful practitioner.

EATING FOR LIFE

Throughout life, conscious eating serves the best interests of your body, mind, and spirit. If, every time you eat, you recall that the food is promoting your health and well-being, you may be adding to its healing power. There is a long tradition of saying grace with meals: blessing the food before it is eaten and giving thanks for receiving it. Today, when we have so little time to even enjoy a meal, we often forget to be thankful for what we are given to sustain us in life. The following story may help you remember.

During World War II, a British officer was captured by the Japanese and put into a concentration camp in Indochina. The food was meager and appalling. Many people died of starvation and malnutrition. Every day, when this officer was given his rations, no matter how sorry an excuse it was for food, he held his bowl up to heaven and offered thanks for all the nutritious food he was receiving, saying that he knew the food had everything it needed to sustain him.

At the end of the war when his camp was liberated, the officer showed no signs of malnutrition or any other deficiency disease. The doctors asked him how he had survived the ravages of such inadequate nourishment. He attributed his health to thanking his Creator for providing him with everything he needed to survive.

Chapter 7

৯Moving for Life

Movement is life. Without movement, we stagnate, wither, and lose our appetite for living. The movement I talk about in this chapter is planned and conscious. We call it exercise, and it is good for the body and the mind. As we exercise, we relinquish, even for a few moments, our minds and let our bodies flow with life energy. Exercise frees mental and emotional energy and allows us to let go of our ideas about how life has to be. In moving, we reconnect with the life force that sustains us, and moves in and through us.

We all need some form of regular exercise at least an hour a day. Your circulation, joints, and mental well-being depend on it. Exercise can retard aging and remove the effects of stress from your body. Exercise also releases energy that accumulates in your auric field. If this energy is not moved, it stagnates and can cause disease.

You can eat more and different types of food when you exercise regularly, because the body needs more fuel. Regular exercise actually allows for carbohydrate tolerance and can ameliorate late-onset diabetes by adjusting the metabolism.

The psychological benefits of exercise are mood elevation, increased self-esteem, and improved memory. It can reduce anxiety and depression considerably. Exercise has a high feel-good factor. You get to be proud of yourself for working out and moving. It also stimulates the release of precious endorphins into your blood, which heightens your sense of well-being. Getting up and moving for an hour can shift the doldrums and help depression.

The form of exercise you choose depends upon what you feel drawn to. For some, it's the slow, graceful movements of yoga, for others it's a quick and energizing aerobic class. You may enjoy walking, bicycling, working out at the gym, attending a regular exercise class with friends, or dancing. As with anything else in your life, balance is important in how you approach an exercise program.

THE NEUROSIS OF COMPULSIVE EXERCISE

Being compulsive about exercise is not a balanced approach and is neurotic. There are people who live in fear of gaining weight or even of dying if they miss a few exercise sessions. Fear should never be the motivating factor in any activity we choose. It defeats the purpose of exercise and is not healthy for the mind/body/spirit. Pleasure is a far superior motivating force, not to mention better for your health. Using pleasure as motivation simply requires tuning into yourself and asking what your body needs and wants now.

Many people believe, unconsciously, that near-starvation eating patterns and strict and punishing exercise programs are their cross to bear for not being good enough. You can always spot people who are compulsive. They have great bodies and faces from hell.

They seldom smile and have that drawn-down quality around their mouths. There is an air of self-punishment about them.

If this description applies to you, take a look at your attitudes about self-worth. Do you feel you are worthy of love, kindness, and respect? Can you begin to heal your pain by treating yourself with that sort of respect and stop taking your self-abuse out on your body? Your body is doing all it can to support you in the best way it knows how. Be gentle and thankful to it for the support it provides you.

TYPES OF EXERCISE

Whatever form of exercise you choose, it should promote fitness, stamina, weight control, and increased lung capacity. Such exercise helps burn calories, energizes the mind/body/spirit, and releases tension accumulated from sitting or standing all day. Let's look at different forms of exercise which may be conducive to your well-being and beauty regime.

Exercise that works on the cardiovascular (CV) system strengthens the heart, lungs, and muscles, and can help regulate blood pressure. Physical fitness instructors recommend up to half an hour of CV exercise as part of any workout program. In the gym, this may consist of walking on the treadmill, cycling, or using the dreaded step machine.

Exercise that works on the skeletal system (weight training and weight-bearing exercise such as brisk walking or running) improves the metabolic functions, nurtures the blood, and builds strength. It can reduce fatigue and increase stamina. This type of exercise is highly recommended for menopausal women who are concerned about osteoporosis. Weight-bearing exercise actually increases bone mass. It also improves physical strength, strengthens tendons and connective tissues, and increases flexibility and strength in the joints, all of which reduce the risk of injury associated with osteoporosis.

I hadn't considered doing weight training until a recent visit to friends in the United States. All my post-menopausal friends were deeply into regular gym programs. I tried it and felt so good that, when I returned to the U.K., I started going to a local gym. I now love working out, and my feeling of strength and stamina is worth the effort. If I am anxious about work or personal issues, working out at the gym helps me to clear my mind of worrisome thoughts and think more lucidly about the problems facing me. For years, my preferred exercise has been yoga, swimming, and hiking. I still love these activities and feel stronger in them as a result of my gym work.

Yoga

Yoga is the ancient form of movement developed in India as part of the Hindu philosophy and religion. It concentrates on developing smooth and graceful movements through stretching and moving the body in coordination with the breath. It stimulates well-being and can rebalance the entire metabolic system. Yoga helps to regenerate the life force and send it through the entire body. Yoga can be done at any age; I have seen teachers in their nineties practice yoga with grace and stamina. It is also an excellent form of exercise for people who are incapacitated or handicapped in some way.

There are numerous types and schools of yoga. I will mention the two types I practice. One is Hatha yoga, in which stretches and breathing are used to open the body to greater flexibility and stamina. Regular practitioners of Hatha yoga attest to never being ill and having great resiliency. This is because Hatha yoga strengthens the immune system through movement and breathing.

Pranayama yoga is the practice of controlled breathing. It can be used to regulate the heart, blood pressure, and digestion. Pranayama yoga is generally done after a Hatha yoga session. Accompanied with meditation, it is deeply calming and stabilizing.

People who practice yoga as a way of life are generally vegetarian and incorporate meditation as part of their practice. Yoga instruction in the West, however, is typically diluted to fit Western capabilities in terms of lifestyle. How far you choose to go with yoga is up to you.

Doing yoga can be a totally cleansing and rejuvenating experience. I have experienced great healing throughout the thirty years I have been practicing yoga. I have also met exceptional people who have committed their lives to teaching and communicating its benefits. Classes are universally available.

Martial Arts

Tai Chi, Shintaido, and Aikido are the three martial arts with which I am familiar. Originally developed as defense techniques in the Orient, they are beautiful forms of movement which inspire grace, intelligence, and awareness. A ninety-two-year-old woman I met recently practices Tai Chi daily and reports that it gives her coordination, flexibility, and mental and physical stamina. Martial arts are taught throughout the West and in every major city in the world.

There are stories about great masters of these arts who, well into their eighties, can challenge their younger students without hesitation. Martial arts are an excellent form of exercise. In addition to providing a rigorous physical workout, they help women overcome the idea of themselves as weak damsels in distress. They build confidence and assertiveness. If you are fearful, inhibited by timidity and shyness, or afraid of expressing aggression, nothing will open you up to your yang or male side quite like a good martial arts class. There, you become one of the boys for an hour. It is a worthwhile experience to punch, chop, and shout, and know that it is all right to do so. Many women love the classes because they can exercise, firm up, and have fun while at the same time safely deal with their aggressions.

Aerobics

The term aerobics generally refers to fast-moving exercises done to music, usually in a group class. The class may be a combination of many forms of exercises, depending on what the instructor chooses to create. Aerobics are designed to raise the metabolic rate, burn off calories, and increase strength, stamina, and lung capacity. This type of exercise is vigorous and can shift your psychophysical energy considerably. When done to good music, with a good stretching session plus some more strenuous exercises, your body feels great. You sweat, loosen up, and move in ways you only dreamed about.

Many women go twice to three times a week for classes and enjoy the experience of working out with familiar faces on a regular basis. Most health clubs and gyms offer these classes. As they are physically challenging, if you have any health considerations, check with your doctor before participating.

The Gym

In gyms with a full range of machines you can have a comprehensive workout and develop long, sleek muscles and a sense of strength that lends confidence and stability to other areas of your life. Women are developing parts of their body that they never imagined would have muscles, and feeling better for it. One woman I know no longer wears shoulder pads because, for the first time in her life, she has shoulders. For another friend, the gym is her answer to jet lag, moodiness, and even the common cold.

Working out needs to be regular for any benefits to accrue. Some physical fitness instructors suggest daily workouts, increasing the sets on each machine over time to build strength and stamina. If you can manage two to three sessions a week, you are winning.

If you do opt for the gym, you must heed the wisdom of the instructors. There needs to be a warm-up period before the stamina exercises and strength work, and then a proper cool-down. This is essential or your muscles will become stiff and hard and you'll walk like those men who spend all day in the gym and look like the Hulk.

Check out your local gym and talk with the people who run it. You need to feel comfortable in order to truly benefit from working out. If you can manage it, I recommend a personal trainer. Try one for a week or two to get you started. His or her advice and motivation techniques can make a difference in how well you use the machines.

Swimming

Swimming is an excellent overall exercise with the entire body stretched and engaged. Doctors recommend it for many physical conditions; it is especially good for rheumatoid arthritis and other joint problems. It increases mobility and is a pleasurable form of exercise. Though it is not aerobic or weight-bearing, it helps increase lung capacity. For full benefit, swimming three to four times weekly is recommended.

Many pools offer aqua-aerobics classes. Doing aerobics in water allows you to exercise your body at a level that is impossible on dry land. Weights and floats help you really work your muscles. Many mature women get strength, stamina, and a terrific sense of well-being from them. After a morning aqua-aerobics class to stimulating music, you feel awake and ready for the day.

Walking and Jogging

These two forms of movement serve the body well, strengthening the lungs and cardiovascular system, provided you don't overdo it. For anyone over 40, jogging needs to be considered in terms of the wear and tear on the joints. Research has shown vigorous walking to be as effective as jogging in getting the pulse rate up and stimulating the breathing.

You get to enjoy more of the beauty around you when you walk and it can be a form of therapy for the mind and spirit. Done regularly, it provides a legitimate form of exercise. If you don't like the idea of walking alone, ask a friend to join you or find a walkers' club. You can vary your walking route, taking trails in parks and in nature, walking to shops or to work. Many people walk to work as a way of getting in their exercise time. If you live close enough to your workplace, you may want to consider it.

Sports

Tennis is a favorite form of sports exercise for many. My seventy-five-year-old aunt has been playing tennis daily for over forty years. She is unhappy if for any reason she has to give up her regular game. It has kept her fit, strong, and sound through the years of running a business, raising a family, and looking after her elderly mother.

It is never too late to take up a sport. I have met many women who started to play their sport after the age of fifty. Check with your doctor if you have any concerns about the rigor of a particular sport. When starting a new form of exercise, you may have aches and pains at first which come from using muscles that have been dormant for years. Massage may be in order for a few weeks to help you over the adjustment period. Also use *Arnica* 6x before and after a sports activity. It is good for relieving muscle pains and aches.

Golf is also popular—those who play regularly claim that the game keeps their minds sharp and bodies fit. Many find the game addictive and find it easy to have this form of exercise become part of their lives.

Whatever sport you choose, take the time to learn it correctly. It will save you frustration and possible despair. Learning a sport is worth the effort.

Taking Responsibility for Your Well-Being

Whatever the physical activity you decide on, remember that you are responsible for your energy and how you invest it. If you put your body through an exercise program, you need to eat properly, rest afterwards, and listen to your physical and emotional requirements.

There are people who are better suited to the quiet rigor of yoga and those who thrive on aerobics and other fast-moving activities. The choice is yours. I am simply suggesting that your life will be different once you start moving and experience the benefits of physical exercise. By exercising regularly in a way you enjoy, you will enhance your life. You will feel better, look better, and love yourself more for giving your body the treat of movement.

Chapter 8

℘ Healing for Life

Ancient people understood that the body responds to love, care, and positive thoughts as well as to the healing properties of natural light and plants. They knew that for any cure to work, the whole person must be treated, not just the site of the illness. The Ancients were able to restore the body's equilibrium with minimal interference. They had rituals and practices that protected the energy system of the body, and cultivated prayer and meditation to strengthen the spirit to prevent emotional fragmentation as well as physical disease.

In our search for solutions to the weakening health that appears to be endemic in the world today, we are beginning to reexamine the hitherto hidden, suppressed, and derided wisdom of the Ancients. This chapter looks at three forms of holistic medicine and the benefits they can offer you. Holistic medicine means that it is natural, considers the working of the mind/body/spirit as the basis of any form of treatment, and uses treatment to restore balance and harmony throughout. All three come from old, time-honored traditions of healing.

The forms of medicine described here (homeopathy, acupuncture, and hands-on healing) are based on philosophic principles which do not vary with time or practice. They don't need to be changed because they work. Homeopathy is now two hundred and fifty years old and has not shifted its philosophy in that time. Homeopaths today still practice along the same lines as past generations of classical homeopaths. Traditional Chinese Medicine, which includes acupuncture and herbalism, has been practiced for over five thousand years. By contrast, Western allopathic medicine has no underlying philosophy. It is forever shifting its ideas about treatment and is often at the beck and call of the pharmaceutical companies and their greed.

The result of the allopathic approach to medicine is an epidemic of weakened immunity seen globally today. People are given drugs from the time they are born. Drugs suppress the immune system by weakening the kidneys, the seat of our immunity. The kidneys and the immune system have to work overtime to filter and process the toxic chemicals in the body. The result is an immune system that crashes easily when too much stress is added to its already burdensome load.

Holistic practitioners, on the other hand, are not like allopathic doctors who give their patients so-called miracle drugs, only to tell them later that there are harmful side effects. When holistic doctors give a remedy or do a treatment, they are not practicing medicine on such shifting philosophical sands. Holistic medicines have a long record of safety and effectiveness for human beings. Unlike allopathy, holistic medicine does not use animals for testing because such research cannot determine how people will react to any given substance.

The three forms of healing covered in this chapter are just a sample of the many types of natural medicine available which can redress dysfunction in the mind/body/spirit. I chose these three because they have been effective in improving my health and well-being. I have trust in the practitioners who follow these disciplines and I respect their medicine. I don't want to be dependent upon doctors who can only offer me drugs or surgical procedures. My choice in medicines has given me health, vitality, and grace.

HOMEOPATHY

I am a registered, classical homeopath and have trained for many years. In the process, I have developed a healthy respect for this natural, life-enhancing medicine. It is safe, gentle, and extremely effective in addressing the imbalances of the human energy system. It works on the physical, emotional, and mental levels to treat human ills. Homeopathy restores balance where there is disharmony and can support people in times of stress, dysfunction, loss, or trauma.

Homeopathy is the treatment of symptoms according to the principle of "like cures like." This means that if a substance can create a symptom in a healthy person, that same substance can be used to treat that condition in a diseased person. I like to use the example of coffee when explaining how homeopathy works. If you were to drink a very strong cup of black coffee, you would probably experience the following symptoms: your hands would start to sweat, you might feel your stomach and bowels churned up, your nerves would make you feel anxious, and you might not be able to sleep until the coffee wore off.

If you came to my clinic complaining of loose bowels, anxiety, insomnia, and excessive sweating, coffee might be one of the 1,500 remedies that I would consider for treating your condition. This is because your symptoms match the symptoms coffee creates in a healthy individual. This is the treatment of like with like.

Homeopathic remedies are made from plant, animal, and mineral matter. They are given in highly diluted quantities so that the quintessential energetic pattern of a substance remains, but not the dangerous alkaloids or poisons which remain in its substantial form. We give a patient a minimal dose of a remedy that has similar properties as his or her condition. Our purpose is to stimulate his or her vital force, that is, his or her immune system, to regain balance.

We wait and watch, observing how symptoms disappear or change after a remedy is given. Homeopathy is slow and it may take time to redress chronic conditions. Yet, it is, in many cases, so complete and effective in its action that a longstanding health problem disappears and does not return. It is extremely fast in addressing acute symptoms such as headache, fever, constipation, diarrhea, shock, colds, and pain.

Homeopathy can be used from birth to death, for the variety of conditions and ailments that exist in the human condition. It is suitable for the elderly because it has no side effects. We use homeopathy for childbirth to assist in a smooth delivery and we also use it throughout pregnancy to build strong tissues in the fetus and to prepare the mother for delivery. It is effective for antenatal bruising, insufficient flow of milk, and other symptoms that occur in babies and new mothers.

Homeopathy can also help women through the transition into menopause, without the use of hormone replacement therapy (HRT), which consists of synthetic hormones, primarily estrogen. HRT can cause cervical and breast cancer. Look carefully at the contraindications that come with any HRT package. Would you even want to tempt fate by putting these synthetic hormones into your body?

Homeopathic estrogen and progesterone, highly diluted, in substantial doses of natural hormones, do the same thing for the body, without the harmful side effects of HRT, including the monthly bleeding which irritates the delicate tissue of mature women. It may surprise you to know that women in the British Royal family have been using homeopathy and this particular form of it for a number of years. Their level of vitality and resistance to age is due, in part, to their use of natural medicine.

Homeopathy has been a staple medicine in the Royal family for five generations. The Queen Mother is the patron of the Royal Homeopathic Hospital in London, and the British National Health Service provides homeopathic treatment. Homeopathy is also practiced extensively in Latin America, India, Australia, and throughout Europe where it originated.

Homeopathy is designed to fit individual cases. That is why homeopaths do not categorically offer a remedy for a condition. We want to know what is special and unusual about your case. You are, after all, an individual and your condition will reflect that. The art of homeopathy is to find the remedy that works for any individual. For instance, we have over 150 remedies for headaches alone. Finding what is particular about your individual headache and supplying the appropriate remedy can cure you of pain and stop recurring symptoms.

Homeopathy is nontoxic. If the homeopath fails to find the remedy that is the correct match for your symptoms (the similimum), that remedy will simply not be effective. You cannot harm a person by giving him or her the wrong remedy. If it is not the similimum, the body quickly eliminates the remedy.

Learning how to self-treat is important in homeopathy for the minor aches and pains that people suffer in the course of a day. All my clients have small first-aid kits with ten widely used household remedies. They administer their own remedies and can treat their families and friends. You can buy homeopathic remedies in health food stores. They are inexpensive and, if taken care of properly, can be kept for years without losing their potency.

For persistent problems which do not respond to self-treatment, constitutional homeopathic practitioners can help with remedies in much higher dilutions than those available in health food stores. They can treat such health conditions as asthma, migraine, menstrual problems, heart disease, and cancer. Homeopathic remedies can also treat depression and other emotional and mental imbalances which allopathic doctors tend to suppress with heavy medication. Homeopathy has the capacity to change a condition, without the side effects of toxic drugs.

If you suffer from chronic and persistent symptoms which limit your life, consider homeopathy. I have seen more healing through homeopathy than I imagined possible. I have witnessed chronic pain cease, difficult children stabilize, and lives become happier.

I would not want to be without homeopathy in this stressful world. It has brought me healing, stability through times of change, rejuvenation, and elimination of fear. Homeopathy has treated my family's predisposition to cancer and lymphatic conditions. Over the years, my health has improved and my mental outlook has improved. I attribute this to extensive homeopathic treatment. What more could you ask of a medicine?

ACUPUNCTURE

Where homeopathy works to shift the biochemistry of the body, acupuncture moves the energy of the body. It restores balance and is sound, effective, painless, and reliable. It, too, can be used for all conditions and problems.

An ancient form of healing which has been practiced continuously in China and the Far East for thousands of years, acupuncture has emerged in the West in the past thirty years and is beginning to be recognized as an effective treatment for a wide range of conditions, including those that conventional medicine has little or no success in treating.

Energetically based, acupuncture works by treating the twelve meridians, or energy channels, that run through the body. These are nonanatomical lines which correspond to function and organs. They are formulated by time of day, seasons of the year, and the elements. Acupuncturists begin diagnosis by listening to the different pulses of the body, which reflect the energetic state of the organs and meridians and indicate where the imbalance lies. Whereas a conventional doctor tests only one pulse, an acupuncturist tests nine and then treats the imbalances with small disposable needles placed at the appropriate acupuncture points to rebalance the energy on a specific meridian.

Like homeopathy, acupuncture listens to and observes the whole person. The acupuncturist looks at your eyes, tongue, and complexion, observes your reactions, and pays attention to your emotional and mental states. The acupuncturist shifts and finetunes the flow of energy along your meridians until balance is restored. This can be accomplished in one session or may require multiple visits, depending on the condition. The acupuncturist may prescribe Chinese herbs in addition to the needle treatment.

Acupuncture has proven useful for many acute and chronic conditions. It has shown itself superior in the treatment of ringing in the ears, arthritis, and congested and blocked organs. Acupuncture can stabilize the liver, tonify the gallbladder, and correct the acidity of the stomach. It is excellent for congestion of the bowels and ovaries and has been used for successful treatment of uterine fibroids and ovarian cysts.

Acupuncture can unblock energy patterns and treat people under high stress. I have used it on several occasions when I felt out of balance and needed a quick solution. I find it particularly helpful during times of grief and change. It can produce astounding results when people are in acute negative states and has even resolved cases considered to be forms of possession.

Acupuncture is now being used as mini-facelifts; the needles being placed to stimulate the points on the face that control sagging muscles and dark rings under the eyes. This tonifying of the muscles of the face can retard the aging process; however, the treatment needs to be done repeatedly over a period of months to be effective.

Restoring balance to a system which is out of harmony can bring beauty, peace of mind, and well-being. Consider acupuncture as a way to redress your health problems. It can work in conjunction with homeopathy, but treatment sessions should not be too close together. They are both powerful tools for healing and should be respected for what they are able to achieve individually.

HANDS-ON HEALING

This form of healing also works along energetic principles, but addresses the chakras, or energy centers. Good healers can shift blocked energy from a chakra and redistribute energy that has been congested or is stagnant. They do so by opening their energy field and directing their energy, thoughts, and prayers to you. They may visualize colors which correspond to your chakras. Hands-on healing can produce some remarkable results.

For the past ten years, I have received this kind of healing from Lady Mary Jardine, who lives and practices in the north of England. She is able to identify blocks in my auric field and addresses the disharmony by directing healing energy into my field. I have experienced the power of her healing on several occasions and am always amazed at what she is able to do when a homeopathic remedy or acupuncture did not help.

When I was in the beginning of menopause and experiencing general confusion and painful heart symptoms, Mary healed me and I regained my strength and stability. The emotional and physical pain diminished and disappeared, and my heartbeat became regular. None of these symptoms recurred, except years later when I was under great stress, and Mary again helped me once more. If I had originally believed that there was something seriously the matter with me, I would have fallen into the hands of the doctors, gone on medication, and become what is known as a cardiac cripple.

There are many hands-on healers who can help weakened systems and fragile personalities. There are now colleges where people who have the gift of healing can train. Barbara Ann Brennan's College of Healing in New York graduates hundreds of healers annually. She is a former bioenergetic psychotherapist with the gift of healing, and her graduates are proficient and well trained.

A good healer can help resolve the roots of physical and emotional problems. They work holistically, looking at the totality of a person's symptoms. Some are able to experience emotional and mental conditions through the gift of second sight and then release many blocks in the energy field. Carolyn Myss trains Medical Intuitives to work alongside doctors to ascertain the underlying psychic cause of illness.

People who practice hands-on healing usually care about humanity and have dedicated their lives to bringing peace and order to ill or out-of-balance people. Their work should be considered valid and useful.

HEALING FOR LIFE

We holistic practitioners often see people who are window shopping for someone to heal them of their ills. They come to me for treatment and leave just as I feel we are making progress. We simply don't offer any quick fixes. Expecting to be fixed by a practitioner is not taking responsibility for your health. Real healing takes time, commitment, and a high level of responsibility and well-being. Holistic practitioners know that all disease is rooted in a fragmentation of body/mind/spirit. If you address a physical problem without looking deeper into the nature of the dysfunction, new and different symptoms will emerge.

Take time to consider your healing program. If you are in good health, you may wish to consider preventative care with homeopathy. If you have problems, you may wish to look into homeopathy, acupuncture, herbalism, or hands-on healing. You need to trust a practitioner in order to make a commitment, so be sure you are comfortable with that person before you start a course of healing.

Whatever you do, be willing to see a treatment through. Take responsibility for your condition and do what you can to find the roots of your condition either in your life or your family history. Look at the mental and emotional components that correspond to your condition. There are many good books which can assist you in this. I recommend the work of Louise Hay, a pioneer in this field, and Carolyn Myss, a medical intuitive. These healers are part of a growing, worldwide healing community.

I urge you to consider the realm of possibilities that holistic medicine can offer you. It definitely expands your options for health and beauty.

Part III

Health and Beauty at the Spa

Chapter 9

℘Loving the Face: Treatments

Noticing another wrinkle around your eyes or mouth can pull your spirits right down. Time etches its mark upon us, and though we cannot turn the clock back, there are things we can do to retard the aging process. Good skin care is now affordable and accessible to everyone who wishes to have a clear, healthy complexion. Fundamentally, there are only four things that need to be done on a daily basis to care for and nourish the skin: exfoliation, toning, moisturizing, and protection.

The cells of our skin are replaced every twenty-one to twenty-eight days. They live under the epidermis, the outer layer of our skin. The live tissue under the epidermis is called the dermis. Blood vessels and nerve fibers run through the dermis, and lymph nodes gather and remove toxins and cellular debris. The health of the dermis determines the state of our skin, which is a direct reflection of the condition of the whole person. If the skin is tired and not absorbing nutrients, the body is likely to be fatigued and unable to process and absorb food as well.

The epidermis is waterproof and acts as a protective barrier against the elements of wind, dirt, dust, and chemical pollution. It is comprised mostly of dead skin cells. Every day new cells are pushing up into the epidermis. The art of beauty care is to feed these new cells and exfoliate or remove the old, dead cells. Exfoliation is the removal of the dead cells by peeling or other techniques such as brushing or polishing the surface of the skin.

Aging occurs when the cells in the dermis lose moisture. Specifically, dehydration depletes the dermis cell walls of their vital components, collagen and elastin, causing the cells to become flat and tight. Beauticians are always trying to plump up these cells with moisture and oxygen, using massage and microcurrent therapy.

Facelifting, a surgical procedure with a high risk factor of general anesthetics, pulls the loose skin tight across the bones. Laser surgery eliminates wrinkles by burning them off the top few layers of skin. Both these techniques may possibly damage the skin severely and permanently. They are mechanical, meaning they don't value the living tissue. As such, they do nothing to care for the skin cells.

The life of the skin is dependent on the time you are willing to spend in health maintenance, lifestyle modification, and general beauty care. In skin care, you are concentrating on maintenance of a living organism. I personally don't want to put my body under a knife or the laser. I am willing, with time and care, to invest in my living cells and give them my love and trust in life. True beauty care needs to be an expression of our belief in life.

YOUR SKIN AND YOUR LIFESTYLE

A beauty therapist can tell if a woman is eating properly, taking drugs or medication, and exercising regularly or not. The skin tells everything—how we love or abuse ourselves, and whether we honor or dishonor the temple of our spirit. Beauty care is an on-going commitment to look after yourself.

People come into a health center or spa wanting instant results. In truth, rest, relaxation, sound eating, and sufficient water intake (at least two quarts daily) make as much difference to the state of your complexion as what you put on your skin. Rich foods, for example, are harder on digestion, and the residue, which can be either assimilated or eliminated, shows up on the skin as blemishes and oil.

Cigarette smoking is probably the single worst thing anyone can do for their complexion. The blood vessels, which normally feed the dermis, become too constricted to supply the cells with nutrients and oxygen. Toxins accumulate. Smokers tend to have a dull, green cast to their faces and fine spider-web lines from skin cells starved of moisture and blood.

Beauty treatments may make you feel good, but they won't help repair your skin from the abuse of smoking, fatigue, poor eating and drinking habits, and stress. I have found that these treatments go a long way to help my skin retain its youthfulness if I also take responsibility for my lifestyle and eating habits. There are a variety of products mentioned below. These are ones that have worked well for me. There is now an entire series of health-oriented products currently on the market worth trying.

Don't expect miracles, but do expect, that with proper care and management, you can achieve good results from the skin treatments I describe in this chapter.

DEEP CLEANSING TREATMENT

Professional skin care treatments usually begin with a deep skin cleansing which opens the skin cells to release anything which clogs and congests the pores. It provides the opportunity for new cells to reach the surface of the skin and to be stimulated so that they can be fed with moisture and nutrients. The skin needs to be cleansed first in order to take in nutrients. The same applies to the body in general. In order for absorption to take place, the body needs to be detoxified of substances which block and impede natural function. It comes down to cellular maintenance, whether it is your complexion or your digestion.

Deep cleansing is done in five stages. First, the skin is cleaned with a cleansing milk to remove makeup and superficial dirt. Next, an exfoliating peel is used on the skin along with hot steam which vaporizes the face and helps open the pores. This is done for ten minutes and is followed by the therapist removing blackheads and pustules from the face. The open clogged pores are full of sebum and, in some serious acne cases, pus. This suggests that the blood needs purifying and detoxifying.

The next step is a gentle and relaxing face massage which stimulates the lymph glands located in the dermis to remove stagnant toxins. The massage helps to drain away any impurities left near the surface of the skin as well. It also tones the muscles and releases tension in the jaw, temples, and forehead. A mask is then applied to soothe and tonify the face, followed by a moisturizer. The skin can now breathe properly. It is recommended to stay out of strong sunlight and drink plenty of water to support the skin in its fresh state. When you have skin treatments, eating nutritious food and drinking a lot of water allows the skin to repair itself more quickly and easily.

Aromatherapy for the Face

A few days after such a deep cleansing, your face is ready to be nourished. A treatment called Aromaplaste by Decleor helps to restructure the cells by feeding them with aromatherapy oils rich in vitamins and minerals. Decleor products are based on phytolactic and aromatherapeutic oils and essences. They can quickly revive the skin.

The Aromaplaste treatment first uses an oil called Angelique, a blend of angelica, chamomile, and geranium essential oils, and oils of avocado, hazelnut, and wheat germ. It is good for dry, dehydrated skin and skin which has lost its tone. Avocado and wheat germ can penetrate into the deeper layers of the dermis and provide excellent moisture and nourishment. Angelica and geranium restore firmness and elasticity to the skin.

This is followed by an essential face balm containing beeswax, oil of basil, chamomile, neroli, hazelnut, and Tonka bean resin. This balm is used for curing minor skin problems caused by oily skin. It cleanses and oxygenates, heals irritation, and dissolves impurities. Afterward, a mask of gauze moistened with a mixture of ground sesame, hazelnut, almond, linseed, and wheat germ is placed on the face for twenty minutes. This is a treatment I like to have on a regular basis, as it does wonders for reviving my complexion.

Sensitive Skin Cold Facial and Intensive Collagen Eye Treatment

These are two treatments done together two days after the nourishing aromatherapy treatment. The Sensitive Skin Cold Facial uses a Thalgo product which is excellent for cooling hot and tired complexions. Thalgo products are made with marine plants and seawater and are easily absorbable into the skin, providing nutrition for new cells. The facial soothes the skin and takes the blotches out, as well as the heat from sunburn. It consists of cleansing, peeling, and a massage. Some beauty therapists use acupressure points to promote relaxation of the face and head. A mask of algae and mint is set on the skin for twenty minutes.

The Intensive Collagen Eye Treatment is from an Italian cosmetic line called Dr. Laura. It uses a collagen mask, rather like Zorro's mask, put over the eyes and held in place with a gel. The eyes absorb the collagen for twenty minutes and the results are startling.

My eyes, in use fifteen hours a day from reading and writing, are usually puffy and baggy. The treatment removes these symptoms for me and the fine lines around my eyes have diminished considerably as well. I recommend it without reservation as a way of treating tired and worn skin around and under the eyes.

COLLAGEN VALE TREATMENTS FOR THE FACE

This is a Thalgo treatment containing marine collagen. First the face is cleansed and exfoliated with a peeling cream. A rich serum of moisturizing gel is applied and then thin strips of collagen, which look like strips of paper, are placed on the face and neck. They are made soluble with a gel and gently massaged into the face with steam vapor, which is like a facial sauna. The treatment is not applied to the eyes.

After the relaxing massage, gentle lifting serum is applied and covered by a mask which reinforces the collagen application. It is left on for twenty minutes. At the end of this treatment, your face is as smooth as a baby's bottom and the fine lines around the mouth seem to have disappeared altogether.

The treatment can be repeated after four days and cumulative results are evident without having to search for them. The skin feels firmer and softer and you know it has been deeply nourished.

REMODEL AND LIFTING FACIAL

This treatment, from Moonlife of Italy, works to replenish the collagen and elastin in the cells of the dermis. It employs strips of collagen and elastin that are activated with a gel and massaged gently into the skin with steam vapor for ten minutes. A lymphatic drainage massage is done on the face and then a lifting agent is applied and gently massaged into the skin. A mask is used to assist its absorption.

When the mask is removed, the skin is firm and feels soft and deeply fed. You can see and feel the glow. I have this treatment done on a monthly basis and when I want to look "up" for an occasion. This and the previous treatment produce highly positive effects and are worth the investment.

AHA INTENSIVE ANTI-AGING TREATMENT

This is an unusual treatment devised by Thalgo for skin with fine lines and pigmentation problems. It works on blotchy patches, dull skin, chloasma, and change of life skin discoloration such as liver spots. It uses alpha hydroxy acids (AHA), up to 7 percent, and is an excellent facial for firming as well as evening your skin tone.

The format uses cleansing and then a special peel containing the AHA fine paper-strip mask, containing replenishing vitamins, minerals, and substances from the sea which are 100 percent pure and natural, is put on the skin with an oxygenated lotion and steam vapor. It is worked into the skin as it melts down.

A replenishing serum, which contains red and black algae and is rich in magnesium, copper, zinc, and amino acids, is then applied. Designed to assist the skin in formulating its own collagen and building up cell walls, the serum is used in conjunction with a skin lotion containing the same ingredients. This is thoroughly massaged into the skin and absorbed over a period of fifteen to twenty minutes.

Afterward, the skin is firm and feels fortified. The skin tone is even and liver spots do appear to be minimized. The results of this treatment last longer for me than all the other treatments.

It is suggested that you avoid the sun entirely to prevent aging and always avoid it directly after any treatment. The sun is a contributing factor in skin discoloration. For those suffering from chloasma, which can develop after hormonal changes in the body such as with pregnancy and menopause, taking vitamin B complex and always wearing sunscreen when outdoors can help.

NO MORE ILLUSIONS IN A BOTTLE

My suggestion is to have one of the above treatments monthly, alternating between them if you are happy with the results. These are the treatments I have discovered that help me. You need, of course, to find the treatments that work best for you and then use them regularly.

I look for honesty and integrity in any treatment I choose. The beauty industry is built on illusion, although there is nothing illusory about the income they derive from people's hopes and pandering to our dreams. It is all promises and unrealistic claims with little results. In our desperation to find a solution to our aging, we believe the hype.

A sane approach is to find out how a treatment is going to help you, if you can rely on it to do the job it says it is going to do, and how often you need to repeat the treatment. There are many new and innovative products on the market that will do one of the four things that skin care demands. However, special treatments, which give the skin an opportunity to breathe, absorb moisture, and retain it, are what you are looking for. You don't have to have an expensive product; you need one that works for your type of skin and gives you the moisture, toning, and protection you need. You can also make your own products with an emulsifier, rose water, and aromatherapy oils. Just make sure that you are getting what you need. You don't want harsh products on your skin or products that fail to protect your face.

Check with your beauty therapist to make sure that a treatment is suited to your skin and will be effective. Be realistic and practical before you invest your hard-earned money and precious time in treatments. You should realize that there is a limit to what can be done.

I believe we all need to give our skin a checkup from time to time either with a beauty therapist or with needed lifestyle modifications. Now that I work out regularly, eat wholesome foods, drink two quarts of water daily, cleanse my skin well, and have skin treatments on a regular basis, I look and feel better than I did twenty years ago when I had all those plump little skin cells but did not appreciate them. Oh, the wisdom of age!

Take the time to invest in a series of treatments designed to revive your skin. It is worth it to find natural products and good therapists who know the skin and can give you good beauty care. If you are on vacation at or near a good hotel that has a beauty salon, check to see what they offer. Many spas and hotels have special relaxation and beauty packages designed to provide a series of treatments to cleanse and nourish the complexion over a week or two. It is a good opportunity to treat yourself well and give your complexion a chance to revive; and you can go home with a plan to bring some care and consciousness into your daily health and beauty management.

What you put on your skin is really not as important as what you put into your body. That will determine the state of your complexion. Organic, fresh food, fresh water, and exercise keep your metabolism flowing and in optimal condition. This will be reflected in the way you look.

How you feel controls the master template of the way you look. You have to be willing to realize who you are and fully appreciate your own magnificence. If you find yourself in situations that don't make you feel good, you might try to look within in order to see where your feelings emanate from. You have the right to be as beautiful and lovely as you can possibly be without the approval of others.

You can retard the aging process using natural products and treatments. You will find that developing and maintaining a regular routine will make those products even more effective. I feel, in honesty, that as long as you use good natural products and maintain a daily routine of cleansing, exfoliating, moisturizing, and protecting your skin, you will get good results. Know your skin type and find the products that will give you the moisture, toning, and protection you need. The general idea, as told to me by several beauty therapists, is to moisturize during the day and feed the skin while you sleep.

Chapter 10

℘Loving the Body: Treatments

Body treatments work along the same principles as skin care. The idea is to stimulate circulation and lymphatic drainage, which, in turn, detoxifies the cells of stagnant lipids and plasma. The treatments I cover here include cellulite treatments, body polish, body wraps, hydrotherapy, and saunas.

Body treatments also induce relaxation and have a high feel-good factor. They are generally combined with a short massage or steam bath to open the pores. They help the body release tension and are good for both skin tone and detoxification.

CELLULITE

Giving the skin the appearance of lumpy cottage cheese, cellulite is a buildup of fat and fluid in the body where tension accumulates—around the joints and muscles. It tends to be prevalent on the thighs, buttocks, arms, and abdomen.

Cellulite is a health as well as a beauty problem. Its presence indicates that the body is not effectively eliminating toxins and burning fat. It suggests that the liver's portal system of circulation is not sufficiently stimulated to do the job of elimination.

If you are serious about trying to eliminate cellulite, you can. There's some discomfort, however. You will need to be vigorous in a program that tunes up your metabolism to help burn off the excess fat. This, along with a wholesome diet, lots of drinking water, massage on a daily basis, and a good attitude, can do much to eliminate the problem. An anti-cellulite diet emphasizes water-soluble foods such as fruits and vegetables and bans fatty and indigestible foods such as sausage, cheese, and candy bars. It is said that cellulite does not respond to diet or even to exercise. I disagree. Eating well, drinking sufficient quantities of water, and exercising regularly do have an effect on eliminating unwanted fatty deposits in the body.

Cellulite also responds well to massage and some topical treatments that use marine plants and ivy extract, both of which help eliminate cellulite. Algae rebalances the acidity level of the skin cells by helping to release fat and stagnant water congesting the interior of the cell. Ivy squeezes the impurities out of the cell. In combination with diet and exercise, you can make your body firmer with more stamina, and can eliminate toxins with greater efficiency. Treatments combined with exercise and the self-massage delineated below can actually reform the shape of your leg.

Another cellulite treatment, the Face and Body Perfector, uses microcurrent, leg wraps, and machine massage which penetrates deeper into the tissue with each massage (see Chapter 11).

Self-Massage for Cellulite

This form of self-massage should not be done on the same day that you are having a cellulite treatment, but on the days after you have had a professional session, which allows the tissues time to mend. Massage the cellulite, using a cupping technique, gently twisting the flesh. Break down the fatty deposits with your thumbs and then rub the area with your knuckles to smooth out the deposits. Brush yourself all over with a loofah for five minutes after the massage, directing your brushstrokes upward toward the center of your chest (at the level of the collarbone) so that the lymph can drain the toxins. Do this first thing in the morning or after a bath for twenty minutes.

Be consistent and try to do this massage daily or when you are not having treatment. If you can persist for at least two weeks, you will have enough incentive to continue. Remember, it works best in combination with diet, drinking water, and exercise. Then you have the support of your entire metabolism working for you.

You can make your own anti-cellulite oil or cream. To a gentle emulsifying cream or olive oil base, add oils of thyme, rosemary, and basil for toning and breaking down fat deposits. I also recommend adding homeopathic *Bellis Perennis* 6x (to stop bruising and alleviate tissue damage), *Arnica* 6x (also for bruising and shock to the tissues), and *Rhus Tox* 6x (to help detoxify the cells). Rose water can be added as a skin softener.

BODY POLISH

A body polish is done with a cream-based product containing an exfoliant. The polish is massaged all over the body to remove dead skin cells, then rinsed off in a warm shower. My skin feels silky and smooth and has a youthful glow after a body polish, which I now do on a regular basis.

You can buy body polishes and do this yourself, but it is a treat to have it done for you occasionally. Brushing the skin with a dry brush, rough cloth, or loofah, as described above, accomplishes the same thing, although without the sheen produced by a body polish. Greek and Cypriot women do a version of body polishing by taking a bottle of olive oil to the beach and rubbing sand and oil on their skin. You can do the same at home using salt and oil instead of the sand. Do it in the tub or shower so you can easily rinse off afterward.

BODY WRAPS

A variety of body wraps are available at health spas. The procedure involves the application over the entire body of creams and gels that stimulate drainage and detoxification, then wrapping the body in plastic and/or cloth to promote perspiration which facilitates detoxification through the skin.

At one spa, I received a body wrap using Thalgo products. To begin with, I was rubbed down with a body plasma gel made of marine plants, designed to stimulate circulation and drainage. The gel also protects the skin from the seaweed and algae body mask which is applied on top of the gel. I was then wrapped in a large plastic sheet, with towels on top of that to create heat, and left to relax and stew in these juices for twenty minutes while my body heated up and toxins were released as I perspired. After twenty minutes, I was tingling all over. I took a shower and was then rubbed down with an anti-cellulite cream made from algae and ivy extract.

I felt lighter after this treatment and had to pee every half hour for the rest of the day. It surprised me how well the wrap worked to detoxify. The treatment demonstrated that detoxification is not only an internal function, but can be accomplished through topical applications as well. A body wrap helps to cleanse the blood and rejuvenates the tissues by getting things pumping and circulating better.

After spending ten minutes in the steam bath to warm me and open my pores, I had a second body wrap. The plasma gel is applied again, topped by a cool, soothing, mint-based body mask. This brings the body temperature down. It is relaxing, cooling, and also promotes drainage and detoxification. At the end of this wrap, I did not feel the same effects as the first. Of the two, I thought the marine algae wrap did the most good. The mint wrap is excellent if you are sunburned or overly hot.

HYDROTHERAPY AND SAUNAS

Hydrotherapy uses water or steam to induce relaxation, soothe and heal aches and pains, and reduce tension. Typical forms of hydrotherapy are Jacuzzis and steam baths. Although a dry heat, saunas produce the same benefits as hydrotherapy.

A bath in a large Jacuzzi with multiple jet-stream massage sprays and aromatherapy oils added to the water can feel like bathing in champagne. With dim lighting and twenty minutes to muse, the bath can help you completely unwind. Many health spas offer this kind of hydrotherapy treatment.

I have come to enjoy the wet heat of the steam bath more than the dry heat of the sauna, but this is simply a matter of personal taste. They warm you up, cleanse the pores, stimulate the circulation, and enhance well-being. Saunas or steam baths are found in most spas, health clubs, and hotels and are a lovely treat, especially in the cold months of winter, when we all need our blood warmed.

They can help you relax and detoxify by sweating your poisons away. In Europe, many people follow a regular routine of a sauna or steam bath weekly.

Too high a heat can be difficult for some people and those with heart problems should check with their doctors before taking a steam bath or sauna. People on blood pressure medication should also consult their doctors, as these hot treatments raise the blood pressure slightly.

Chapter 11

℘ᴧNonsurgical Lifting Treatments

I have investigated nonsurgical face and body lifting treatments over the past five years. They involve the use of microcurrent to stimulate the dermis, or deep layer of live skin cells where lymph, blood circulation, and nerve fibers function.

When I considered how far I was willing to go in beauty treatment, the application of microcurrent was the outer limit. I am not interested in any form of treatment that involves injection of animal matter into my body, drugs, anesthesia, or cutting. This eliminates some of the popular current treatments such as collagen implants, laser treatment, or facelifting. For me, microcurrent still falls within the boundaries of good health. In my opinion, these other treatments do not.

In addition to microcurrent, which I discuss below, another nonsurgical lift uses alumina silicate powder to abrade skin wrinkles. With aluminum linked to Alzheimer's disease, I don't want to be exposed to it any more than I have to. Having changed my deodorant to one without aluminum and replaced all my aluminum cooking utensils, why would I expose my face to it? The fine particles can be inhaled all too easily. I don't consider this a healthy treatment.

MICROCURRENT LIFTING

Microcurrent has been used for the past twenty years in medical treatments. As a nonsurgical lift, microcurrent stimulation of circulation and lymph drainage in the dermis increases the efficiency of nutrient absorption and at the same time speeds up the elimination of waste impurities which clog and congest the cells.

The best treatment I have found is the Face and Body Perfector. The recommended Perfector course is ten microcurrent treatments over two to three weeks and a booster treatment monthly to keep up the effects. A conductive gel, rich in nutrients and vitamins, is first applied to create a medium for the current to flow through to the skin. Two gentle probes are then used to conduct the microcurrent into specific muscles. The current is minuscule and cannot be felt. You don't get a sensation of being fried or nuked by this machine. The flow of current varies with each of the stages of treatment, but is gentle throughout.

During my trial course, even with the stress of my daily life, seeing patients, doing workshops, and writing books, I still managed at the end of the day to have some "up" energy in my face rather than the usual sag which is disheartening. I was so impressed I bought the microcurrent machine for home beauty care. It is an expensive machine, but when I added up the number of nonsurgical lifts I had invested in over the past five years, it made financial sense to buy one. This machine is made in Britain and sold universally.

Perfector has been researching with different combinations of current frequency and wave formation to determine which ones penetrate to the dermis better and do the job of stimulating tissues to plump out the cells. The word *plump* is used universally in the beauty industry to describe what happens to flat, tight skin cells after a treatment. The industry is always on the lookout for anything that plumps the cells, and this treatment gets high marks for plumping. In other words, it works.

Basically, the Face and Body Perfector is a salon in a box with nine treatments currently on their system. These include Face and Body Lifting, Cellulite and Stretch Marks treatments, Skin Enhancement, and Purikiss Detoxifying Facial treatment. The Perfector company trains their therapists well in operating the machine properly. Ongoing research and development on their line of face-care products ensures quality to clients and beauty salons, who are the main purchasers of the equipment. For these reasons and the quality of the product, I view the Perfector as a superior microcurrent treatment.

There are treatment programs in the Face and Body Perfector to suit all ages and skin types. Perfector stresses that their treatments are both preventive and corrective, so they can be used by people of all ages. These programs are designed for skin firming, which closes the pores, diminishes fine lines and wrinkles, and smoothes the appearance of the skin. The treatments improve color by increasing circulation. The increased flow of blood to the surface of the skin is excellent for reducing skin discoloration.

Face Perfector Treatments

In the Face Lifting program, the probes conduct the microcurrent into specific face muscles which they then lift and tone.

The Skin Enhancement Program doesn't involve lifting the

muscles. It is excellent for younger skin and helps maintain good tone and a youthful appearance. For more mature skin, it works to eliminate that sallow complexion we are prone to get with illness or too much stress. It also works to open pores and seems to have a good effect on blemished skin; I recommend it for acne and scarring.

A series of treatments can help detoxify the skin and restore normal circulation in problematic skin conditions. Three one-hour sessions at weekly intervals is the recommended course for the Facial Enhancement program. Taken as a single session, it is good as a facial or if you need a pick-me-up. To get the maximum from these treatments, however, it is suggested that you invest in a ten-series course which can really reeducate the skin.

Body Perfector Treatments

The Perfector machine not only gives your face and complexion a new glow, but it can also lift and firm your body. It works on the hands, buttocks, thighs, breasts, abdomen, and upper arms. Microcurrent treatments do not cause weight loss. They tighten and firm the muscles and address the flab and sag that come with age. Even with regular exercise, this can be a problem. Unless you submit to the knife or liposuction, microcurrent is your best bet for helping to firm these muscles. It is especially effective in combination with diet and exercise.

The number of treatments depends on skin condition, age, and lifestyle. As a general guide, six sessions are recommended for the thirty to forty age group, twelve sessions for the forty to fifty age group, and eighteen sessions for those over fifty. An additional six sessions are recommended for smokers and those who have abused their skin with too much sun exposure and poor diet (this includes alcohol, coffee, and tea drinkers). As with other therapies, results are best when treatment is combined with a healthy diet, exercise, and at least two quarts of water a day. Observing an anti-cellulite diet adds to the benefits; this consists of an abundance of fruit and vegetables and a minimal quantity of sugar and fat.

It is best to work on one area of the body at a time. For example, if you want to firm up your thighs, you would have a microcurrent treatment on that area every two to three days for two or three weeks. You could also add anti-cellulite self-massage, giving special attention to your thighs (see Chapter 10).

Perfector Treatments Work
While Perfector treatments are not miraculous, they work. One beauty therapist told me that one of her clients, a woman in her mid-sixties, was scheduled for a facelift. The woman was so pleased with her Perfector treatment that she canceled the surgery.

The effectiveness depends on how willing you are to take responsibility for your health and beauty care. If you abuse yourself with smoking, drinking, lack of sleep, and poor diet, microcurrent treatments are not going to make up for the resulting damage. For those who observe healthful practices, however, Perfector treatments are a good investment in yourself. They give your face the stimulation it needs for drainage, detoxification, and toning. Microcurrent works well in combination with skin care treatment, particularly the deep cleansing, nourishing, and collagen treatments described in Chapter 9.

When you consider that a facelift costs between $10,000 and $15,000 and leaves you looking stretched and slightly unnatural (I can always tell if a face has been surgically lifted), Perfector treatments are a small investment for your face and body care.

Treatments can be as low as $50 and as high as $100, depending on where your beauty salon is located. (See the Resources section for the Perfector company contact information; they can tell you who provides treatments in your area.) Though costly compared to facials and other ways of maintaining your skin, I personally think these treatments are worth it. For me, the microcurrent machine is a serious investment in my anti-aging campaign to look and feel as good as I can for the rest of my life.

Chapter 12

The Finishing Touches: Hair, Makeup, and Nails

What most women consider the primary beauty care treatments in their lives, I regard as the finishing touches. What you do to your hair and makeup is what people see, but it is in fact only a small part of your health and beauty care program.

HAIRCUTS, HAIR CARE, AND COLOR

A good hair style can do wonders for you. The shape of your face and quality of your hair is uniquely yours. If you insist on a hair style that is better suited to a different facial shape and hair texture, you are engaged in a struggle to be someone you are not. Learning to accept your appearance and knowing how to enhance it are part of the skill of expressing your beauty. If you have curly hair, why spend hours and a small fortune trying to straighten it? Why not accept what you have? Enhance what is natural to you and embellish it, if you want to, with highlights or an excellent cut.

You may have a face that looks good with long, curly hair, or one that is better suited to short, cropped hair. You need to know what your options are. It is worth taking some time with a good hairdresser and exploring the styles which look good on you. I had kept the same hairdo for twenty years when I went to a hairdresser and spent a few weeks letting her play with my hair. She put it up, brushed it off my forehead, gave me bangs. She brought out styles that completely changed my vision of myself. Able to look at myself differently, I could see what suited me. The styles were not difficult to create; I could do them myself with a bit of mousse and a hairdryer. As someone who doesn't like fussing, it was perfect for me.

Women today wear their hair in styles that run the gamut from very short to very long. We aren't confined to rigid hair styles that take lacquer or pins to hold them in place. Most of us want something that is easy and manageable, but still looks good. We have a lot of options.

Again, it is harmony we are striving for. Your hairstyle shouldn't overshadow you. If it does, it isn't right for you. *You* need to be seen, not the hair style. The same is true for clothes. If you get a spectacular dress or suit and people don't see you when you wear it, it isn't the right outfit for you.

Taking care of your hair is important. Like your skin, your hair reflects the state of your health. You may notice when you have been ill or under a lot of stress that your hair becomes flat and lifeless. This can be remedied with holistic health care, good food, nutritional supplements, and rest. My hair is alive when I am well and happy.

As a homeopath, I see many people whose scalps are dry and flaky or whose hair is falling out, often due to stress. Over the past ten years, I have treated numerous women with alopecia (hair loss). It is partly a metabolic condition in which nutrients are not being assimilated properly. There is too much fat in the body as a result of it not being digested and eliminated. These women do well on homeopathic treatment and, within weeks, their hair growth is usually restored to normal.

Homeopathy works better than any topical treatment I know. There are, however, hair treatments that can be used to fortify and nourish the hair. A wide variety is available at salons and pharmacies. You can also use coconut oil, olive oil, or a homemade mixture of mayonnaise and soy sauce as hair treatment. Some women use beer to give their hair body, others sleep with conditioner on their hair overnight. The latter is excellent because it gives the hair time to absorb the nutrients.

If your hair has been overexposed to the sun or pollution, or if you have colored your hair for a long time, a good conditioner, or hair mask as they are now called, will help revive your hair. Hair can only take so much abuse and needs care to keep it healthy. If your hair does not respond to conditioning, consult a homeopath or herbalist. They have remedies to address the imbalance in your biochemistry. If your hair is sick, at some level so are you. Whatever you put on your hair will have no effect until you get healthier.

In the United States and Europe, there is considerable societal pressure on older women to dye their hair to cover its natural gray and look younger. If you have come to the point in your life when you are considering dying your hair, please remember that hair dye is carcinogenic. One of the first pieces of advice doctors give people with cancer is to stop dying their hair.

If you are determined to do this, I suggest using semi-permanent colors which aren't so toxic. Hair specialists often suggest that you pick a lighter color than your natural one. Darker hair makes the skin look sallow. It has been my observation that hair dye usually makes women look older because of the contrast of vibrant hair color with aging skin. The face then needs constant makeup to match the high tones of the hair.

To accept your age and the process of aging is magnificent. This is an uphill battle for most women, however. Many prefer to endure the annoyance of putting a rinse or hair color on their hair and the anxiety of watching for gray roots to show. I recommend that you think carefully. Can you visualize yourself with silver threads that show the world your age? Can you imagine yourself with a different color of hair that is lighter, more in harmony with your skin tone?

Look in a mirror and ask yourself what is important to you. What do you want to say to the world? Is looking natural important? Is being youthful important? Can you keep a youthful image up without too much work? The answer to the last question is the clincher for me. Once the beauty measures start cutting into my time and money, I lose interest quickly.

I colored my hair with henna until it became serious work to cover the increasing areas of gray. I got rid of the dyed hair by telling my hairdresser to cut it very short. (It took two years for it to grow to its usual length.) I am glad I dared to do it. I love the silver quality of my hair now. It is healthy and vibrant and suits me. I do understand that this is an important decision for every woman to make and I hope that you approach it with forethought and grace.

MAKEUP

There are many guides to selecting the right color for your complexion and applying it, so I won't spend time covering what every beautician can tell you. I would like to say something in favor of makeup, however. Makeup protects the skin against sun, chemicals, and dirt and acts to enliven the face. It is a wonderful aid for times when you are less than optimally beautiful.

I love makeup and am always at the cosmetics counter looking at new lines, sampling brands, and having that free makeover when companies are promoting their products. I am also enough of an artist to appreciate the way different people put the slab on my face. Makeup lends fascination, authority, and elegance and has the ability to highlight the good points and diminish the poor ones.

Color and application are fundamental to a proper job. Makeup foundation should always be a shade lighter than your natural skin tone so that you don't have a line on your jaw or at your neck. You can blend two, even three different foundations to achieve the color you want and mix some moisturizer into the blend as well. This helps it to lie on your skin better and gives it some moisture for later in the day.

Powder can be brushed or patted on with a puff to give the face a finished and matte look. Lightly does it with powder. Too much looks like you are filling in the cracks, and we all know this is the last image we want to create.

Blusher can be lightly applied to the side of the cheekbone and up to the corner of the eye. It gives the face a shadowing that highlights the bone structure and also adds color, which many women need.

Professional TV and film makeup artists mist the face with water when they finish applying powder and blush. This sets the makeup so that it doesn't crawl or run in heat or with perspiration and enables it to stay on the face without turning color or becoming saturated in face oil. It is a good tip if you work all day and don't have time to redo your face. It is also good for travel or evenings when you are out for long periods of time.

Highlighting the eyes and lips gives the face definition. The degree to which you apply these items should be appropriate to the occasion and to the time of day. It looks funny to see overly made-up women during the day or looking drab and lifeless at a party at night.

As we mature, finding makeup that doesn't hide in the cracks is important. A highly refined makeup is the answer, but be sure to test it first. A professional beautician can be of real service here. As we age and the fine lines develop, we risk having our makeup look like a trowel job. It is not becoming or necessary. Better no powder than the trowel.

Lip liner helps to define the shape of the mouth and can cover up flaws. One beautician gave me a tip that I have used ever since. Use a dark lip liner on the outside of the lips, a lighter lip liner to fill in the lips, and apply a gloss color on top of this. Done in this way, the lipstick almost never has to be reapplied. The lips stay colored and attractive all day long.

My personal feeling about makeup is that it makes a woman attractive. There are few women over forty who have the face and skin to get away without makeup. It doesn't mean you have to wear it all the time, but, especially in winter when our complexions are sallow and drab, makeup is a healthy-looking boost. In the summer, it may be less essential.

Finding the balance with makeup is the important thing. Looking painted is not attractive and looking washed out is equally bad. It is worth learning how to use makeup and deciding what and when you want to wear it.

Using natural organic makeup has become an issue since recent studies indicate that cysts removed from the breasts of women with cancer have been encased in lipstick and makeup. It is important to find a makeup line, such as Gabrielle or other organically based products, which do not use chemicals that can have a dangerous effect on your health. Many of these organic lines are beautiful and carry a guarantee that they are harmless to your health and well-being.

NAILS

Nail care is a big beauty item for many women. I have never let anyone work on my hands, so it was a bit traumatic to have my nails done for this book. It turned out to be an enjoyable experience, however. The manicurist who worked on me applied paraffin wax to my hands, wrapped them in plastic, and then put them into cotton mitts for twenty minutes. To my surprise, my hands emerged soft and lustrous. This strikes me as a lovely way to preserve the quality of good skin on the hands. It is nourishing to the skin and felt wonderful afterward.

Looking after your hands and nails is a way of retarding the aging process. Hands show age more readily than the face. Skin lotion and a good manicure from time to time is a simple way of looking after your hands. Many women have their nails done regularly and even have extensions and false nails put on. Nails that are too long and varnished have always reminded me of claws. It is part of the artifice of our sex, but I don't find it attractive and even regard it as a bit frightening. Such nails put me off wanting to come close to the person. Again, it is a question of personal taste.

Dirty and ragged nails are not attractive. The message they send to me is that beauty doesn't count for that person. Having well-shaped and clean nails is important for grooming. However, the degree of adornment and color you want to add is up to you.

Part IV

Health and Beauty
in the Home

Chapter 13

✒ A 21-Day Program for Regaining Health and Beauty

The idea for this program emerged when I had a three-week holiday to revive, rejuvenate, and heal between work assignments. I was tired, fragile, and worn out from too much stress. I gave serious thought to what I wanted to do for myself on all levels, from the spiritual to the physical. The plan detailed here served me well and I would do it again, given the time and money. You can alter it to suit you and your needs. It can be done at home or away on vacation. The first time I went through this program was on the Mediterranean island of Cyprus, staying at a monastery and visiting a day spa for treatments.

Before I began my three-week break, with the intention of focusing on my health, I consulted my homeopath and was given a constitutional treatment which would help revive my energy. The consultation took an hour and gave me an opportunity to review my health on all levels.

I then went to a health food store and selected the vitamin supplements and detoxification program I felt I needed. I knew it was one of those special times to take supplements to attempt to revive my depleted body. I chose an herbal-based detoxification program which incorporated psyllium seed husks for cleansing the bowels and three different herbal tinctures to stimulate the liver and lymph system. The herbs, in liquid form, were to be taken twice daily with water.

The other supplements I selected were garlic tablets for blood purification, euphrasia tablets for my eyes, a liver tonifier, a menopausal vitamin supplement, and dandelion and goldenseal to strengthen my immunity. I also bought herbal tinctures of melissa and passiflora to calm and soothe my nerves, which were definitely frayed from overwork, and to help me sleep well. Homeopathic *Thymus* 6x would also fortify my immune system (taken for one week). Armed with a supply of supplements, I then bought some good hair conditioner, beauty masks, and herbal teas.

I started my spiritual rejuvenation with a regular program of daily meditation. Each morning upon waking, I lit a candle and some incense and meditated for twenty minutes to half an hour. This was how I wanted to begin my day and end it. However, at night I usually fell asleep before I got to meditation.

I brought notebooks for writing affirmations and did my visualizations every day while floating in the sea. There is something about floating, perhaps the release of gravity, that frees us from reality's pull and allows us to kindle our imaginations to work on our behalf. While floating, I also did my breathing work, using a snorkel (see Chapter 5).

Whenever emotions came to the surface that needed releasing, I would have a short weep and allow myself to hear the truth about my feelings. I didn't indulge them, but I felt it was important to recognize them. I mothered myself, allowing my feelings to be soothed gently and with pure thoughts of love and kindness. In this process, I was learning to let the wounded child have her say, as part of my emotional healing.

I fasted on fruit for the first three days and then added raw vegetables, some fresh fish, and white cheese. I made salads daily from the local fresh produce and invested in a grater for grating carrots and cucumbers. I ate a lot of fresh garlic, lettuce, tomatoes, carrots, cucumbers, radishes, and onions. I added olives and almonds to this when I wanted them. This was the best diet I could give myself. I enjoyed the local produce and appreciated that nearly everything I was eating was fresh and not grown with chemical fertilizers.

I drank at least two quarts of water each day. When I wanted a change, I drank herbal teas. I was fortunate that fresh juices were sold locally and I could buy grape, peach, and pineapple drinks when I was in need of extra energy, such as before I went to work out or for a long walk. I bought kefir and kombucha tea from a local supermarket and mixed them with grape or passion fruit juice for a delightful drink. If I had available extra weight in my luggage, I would have brought my juicer and made my own juices. I know women who have done this and admire them for their tenacity. I bought olive oil, honey, and carob syrup from the local stores. The oil I mixed with aromatherapy oils such as rose, jasmine, neroli, and lemon and massaged myself with it every day. I also used it for hair treatments and on salad. The carob syrup is used locally for a sweet drink and is a natural cure for constipation. It is similar to fig syrup and tastes delicious. I used it when I wanted something sweet and to assist with elimination.

I made a point of doing the cellulite self-massage (see Chapter 10) daily for twenty days to see if this actually worked to diminish my thighs. In fact, it did make a difference and has since become a habit. I used a small loofah mitt to rub down my body with each massage. I also went through a lot of moisture cream to keep my skin from drying out from the sun, and used a sunscreen that both protected and moisturized. The latter is made by La Prarie and I use it now in my daily life, applying it over my moisturizer.

Each day, I did a 1 1/2 hour workout at the hotel gym. It was not easy to start, but once I got into it and found myself becoming thinner, stronger, and more fit, it became the highlight of my day. I loved the challenge, especially when everything else in my life was so peaceful and calm. It helped me to meet my aggression and anger about things head on. I worked with a trainer for the first few days until I felt comfortable using the gym equipment. Every afternoon after a good half-hour swim and snorkel session in the sea, I took a book to the beach and lay under an umbrella, reading and dozing.

When I arrived for holiday, I already had a good haircut and had been told by my hairdresser to tie my hair up so it wouldn't get sun-bleached and damaged. I used a hot olive oil pack on my hair weekly. For this, I rubbed in the olive oil, tied my hair up with a scarf, and let it soak in, sometimes for two days. Then I shampooed it and applied a hair pack or conditioner. Afterward, my hair was soft and lustrous.

Every day after working out, I had a beauty treatment. One day I got a face treatment, the next day a body treatment (see Chapters 9 and 10). These treatments improved the quality of my skin and taught me a great deal about what works for me. I discovered what I wanted to continue to invest in for my skin and beauty care. The care and attention in the treatments was healing in itself. It was lovely to be pampered.

If you live near a salon or hotel with a spa, you may want to have treatments on a regular basis. You can also improvise on your own at home. I made a facial of avocado and honey occasionally during my three weeks. An Israeli woman in her sixties who had the loveliest complexion I have ever seen gave me this recipe: half an avocado and one large tablespoon of honey applied as a mask for half an hour daily. If you don't eat it off, wait and see how soft it makes your skin.

For a firming mask, you can use a recipe taught to me by European women who would apply this every Saturday afternoon around the pool before their elegant dinner parties. Separate the yolk and white of one egg. Add one teaspoon of olive oil to the yolk, mix together, and put on the face, neck, chest, and hands. Whisk the egg white into stiff peaks and apply it on top of the yolk. Let the mask dry for twenty minutes. Don't smile or talk or you'll crack it. Wipe it off and feel how firm and tight your face is. Moisturize with a light lotion afterward.

I made a point of getting a good night's sleep and was generally in bed by 9 P.M., reading for an hour before falling into blissful sleep. I slept till 8:00 each morning and took some time to think about my dreams which were rich and interesting. Having the time to reflect on your dreams awakens your inner ear.

I followed this routine each day and watched the tension drop away. I saw my body lose fat and flab from the workout, self-massage, and cellulite treatments. I felt revived by not having to do anything but look after myself and listen to my inner guidance.

I loved my books and the gentle pace of my day. It was a blissful experience. It taught me that I could recover my health and find my beauty. It was time and money well invested in myself. I understood that it was okay to enjoy this healing period. I left Cyprus feeling like a new woman and determined to keep up the workouts, the water drinking and good eating, and some face and body care treatments.

I knew I never again wanted to be as tired, strung out, or worn down as I was when I arrived on Cyprus. Clearly, that meant I would have to keep some firm boundaries in my life, not take on more than I could reasonably deliver, and take time each day, each week, and each month for the things that give me pleasure and happiness and support my beauty and health.

Times of rejuvenation are essential. They help shift the focus of our lives when we are in need of healing. This type of program on holiday or when you have the time to indulge yourself reminds you how responsive your body/mind/spirit is to positive input and conscious care. The body loves touch, good, wholesome food, and lots of water and exercise. The mind loves tranquillity, beauty, and peace, and the spirit is simply happy and content to be recognized and honored. Providing all of this is the path to beauty.

This program works if you apply it in your life. You can even do a lot of these things as part of your daily practice whether you are working or having a rest. They are essential principles for health and well-being. If you apply them on a regular basis you will be less likely to use them for emergency repair service when you are worn out and in need of rejuvenation.

Investing in your healing is worth it only if you know that you are worthy of the beauty, health, and healing you know you deserve. If you want to look and feel well, the investment of time, energy, and money will serve you.

HOMEMADE REMEDIES FOR BEAUTY CARE

You can make many of your own potions for beauty care. I use my own mixtures, rather than invest a minor fortune on products, and find them excellent for my needs. Frankly, I find that my complexion responds as much to what I put *into* my body in terms of good, wholesome food, natural herbal teas, and spring water. I also know I look my best when I have had plenty of rest. There is no product that can match this medicine.

When I make up my own face care products I search for the best natural oils and products. I mix them in glass containers which protect against light. I suggest finding either blue or brown glass jars or bottles. They will preserve your product for longer.

Tonics

These can be made from pure spring water mixed with oils of jasmine, peppermint, rose, neroli, and lavender. You can make a stimulating tonic for daytime use with peppermint, neroli, and jasmine. A calming tonic can be made with lavender and rose. Dilute the essential oil to the strength that appeals to you and add only small quantities of oil to give you the effect you desire. One to two drops of an essential oil is sufficient.

Face Creams

I make up a mixture of face cream that I use both for daytime use and at night to nourish my skin. I live in a very arid part of the country and skin care needs supplementing often.

I use jojoba oil as my carrier base because it is most like the skin's natural oils. I add to that:

- ✧ oil of rose, neroli, and lavender
- ✧ a drop of vitamin E oil
- ✧ Arnica oil, calendula, and hypericum oil (one drop of each)

This mixture gives my face nourishment and healing substances that repair and keep wrinkle formation to a minimum.

If I find that my skin looks tired and needs a lift I will use a cream made from calendula, mint, and rose oils. I will use the egg facial mentioned earlier (see page 172) and place a drop of this mixture onto my skin before applying the mask. This gives my face a glow and is excellent for use before a big occasion when you want to look your best.

I use these mixtures daily and feel that consistent care with cleansing, exfoliating, and nourishment keep my complexion looking good. When I go off my routine, I find that my skin becomes blotchy and begins to look fatigued.

You can also melt down bee's wax and add olive oil to any of the oils mentioned to create a salve that will feed your skin. The lighter this lotion, the less it is likely to clog your pores and be assimilated into the skin while you are resting.

If you are not able to find liquid medicated potencies, you can dissolve a few homeopathic tablets in water and add that to your mixture.

Afterword

THE GESTALT OF BEAUTY: BEAUTY IS GREATER THAN THE SUM OF ITS PARTS

Anything you do to improve your appearance and feel good about yourself comes from an intention to be attractive and happy. That intention is not about the perfection of your skin, makeup, hair, or nails, nor is it about whether you are overweight or underweight. The intention to express your beauty and let your spirit shine out into the world comes from your desire to be the best that you can be.

Allowing your spirit to shine means accepting that who you are goes well beyond any singular or collective attempt to be beautiful, but comes directly from the experience that you are beauty itself. You are simply going to tidy up the bits that may be a bit raggedy and give some attention to presenting your true self.

We are all goddesses at heart, and I know that you know this about yourself. Whatever stops you from allowing this to be expressed needs to be harvested out. Attitudes which limit your being and suppress your expression don't serve you any longer. Holding grudges against your parents, siblings, classmates, old boyfriends, ex-husbands, or partners will only bring you down a notch. Do you really need or want that? Isn't your beauty ready for the world? Does it truly matter what your age, size, skin color, or sexual preference is? I don't think so.

What I do know is that it is definitely time to let your beauty shine. Be yourself, not a carbon copy of someone on TV or in the films. What is beautiful and unique about you is what will attract the people and experiences to you that confirm and honor you. When you hide behind conventional images of beauty you suppress yourself.

Knowing that you are worthy of love, kindness, and respect, no matter what, is the greatest learning there is in any spiritual practice, religion, or teaching. If you are not living from the place where you know this about yourself, it is time to make a shift in your thinking and begin the healing process by accepting that who you are is love, light, freedom, and beauty itself. Taking the rest of your life to integrate this fully is a spiritual practice. Loving yourself unconditionally and learning how to love others in the world around you is the lesson of life.

I wish you all healing, health, beauty, and the deepest acceptance of who you are. I know when you realize your worth, the world will be illuminated by your grace.

Resources

Alternative Health Resources

Acupuncture Center of Boulder and Chi Kung School at the Body–Energy Center
James MacRitchie and
  Damaris Jarboux
2730 29th St.
Boulder, Colorado 80301
Acupuncture Center: (303) 442-2250
Chi Kung School: (303) 442-3131
fax: (303) 442-3141

Decleor, USA, Inc.
  (information about aromatherapy)
500 West Ave.
Stamford, Connecticut 06902
tel: (800) 722-2219
fax: (203) 967-2680

National Center for Homeopathy
tel: (703) 548-7790

Products

Face and Body Perfector
Burnham, Bucks SL1 7JH, U.K.
tel: 01628-660123
fax: 01628-660100

Spas

Coral Beach Hotel
Coral Bay Hotel and Resort
P.O. Box 2422
8099 Paphos, Cyprus
tel: 357-6-621601
fax: 357-6-621752
e-mail: coraisis@coral.com.cy

Enchantment Resort
525 Boynton Canyon Rd.
Sedona, Arizona 86336
tel: (520) 282-2900
reservations: (800) 826-418
fax: (520) 282-9249
www.arizonaguide.com/enchantment
e-mail: enchant@sedona.net

Ambika offers long term, committed training programs called "Lifechanges with the Chakras" where people find their inner radiance and outer beauty. Contact her at (877) 774-1812 for information.

BOOKS BY THE CROSSING PRESS

OTHER BOOKS BY AMBIKA WAUTERS

Chakras and Their Archetypes: Uniting Energy Awareness and Spiritual Growth

Linking classic archetypes to the seven chakras in the human energy system can reveal unconscious ways of behaving. Wauters helps us understand where our energy is blocked, which attitudes or emotional issues are responsible, and how to then transcend our limitations.

$16.95 • Paper • ISBN 0-89594-891-5

Healing with the Energy of the Chakras

Chakras are swirling wheels of light and color—vortices through which energy must pass in order to nourish and maintain physical, emotional, mental and spiritual life. Wauters presents a self-help program intended to give you guidelines and a framework within which to explore and understand more about how your energetic system responds to thoughts and expression.

$14.95 • Paper • ISBN 0-89594-906-7

Homeopathic Color Remedies

Color has been known to have a strong influence on people and treatment with colored light has been used in naturopathic circles for several decades. Wauters' homeopathic color remedies serve as medicine for our energy body, increasing the energetic flow physically, emotionally, and mentally.

$12.95 • Paper • ISBN 0-89594-997-0

LifeChanges with the Energy of the Chakras

When we face up to the reality of change, we learn to accept its challenges with grace and renewed grit. We can alter our old movies-our old patterns-and gain insights into our nature. We then can be released from the past and find new, healthy options for our lives.

$14.95 • Paper • ISBN 1-58091-020-3

To receive a current catalog from The Crossing Press
please call toll-free, 800-777-1048.
Visit our Web site: **www.crossingpress.com**